TECHNICAL REPORT

Examining Child Care Need Among Military Families

Susan M. Gates, Gail L. Zellman, Joy S. Moini

with

Marika Suttorp

Prepared for the Office of the Secretary of Defense

Approved for public release; distribution unlimited

NATIONAL DEFENSE RESEARCH INSTITUTE

The research described in this report was prepared for the Office of the Secretary of Defense (OSD). The research was conducted in the RAND National Defense Research Institute, a federally funded research and development center sponsored by the OSD, the Joint Staff, the Unified Combatant Commands, the Department of the Navy, the Marine Corps, the defense agencies, and the defense Intelligence Community under Contract DASW01-01-C-0004.

Library of Congress Cataloging-in-Publication Data

Gates, Susan M., 1968-
    Examining child care need among military families / Susan M. Gates, Gail L. Zellman, Joy S. Moini.
      p. cm.
    Includes bibliographical references.
    ISBN-13: 978-0-8330-3902-6 (pbk. : alk. paper)
      1. Families of military personnel—Services for—United States. 2. Child care—United States.
  I. Zellman, Gail. II. Moini, Joy S. III. Title.

UB403.G37 2006
362.71'208835500973

                                                  2006032200

The RAND Corporation is a nonprofit research organization providing objective analysis and effective solutions that address the challenges facing the public and private sectors around the world. RAND's publications do not necessarily reflect the opinions of its research clients and sponsors.

RAND® is a registered trademark.

Published 2006 by the RAND Corporation
1776 Main Street, P.O. Box 2138, Santa Monica, CA 90407-2138
1200 South Hayes Street, Arlington, VA 22202-5050
4570 Fifth Avenue, Suite 600, Pittsburgh, PA 15213-2665
RAND URL: http://www.rand.org/
To order RAND documents or to obtain additional information, contact
Distribution Services: Telephone: (310) 451-7002;
Fax: (310) 451-6915; Email: order@rand.org

Preface

The Department of Defense (DoD) supports the largest employer-sponsored system of high-quality child care in the country. Through accredited child development centers (CDCs), family child care (FCC) homes, youth programs, and other after-school programs, the DoD provides care to over 174,000 military children aged 0 through 12 years. Still, DoD policymakers remain concerned that the system falls short of meeting the needs of military families with children. In a 1992 report, *The Potential Demand for Child Care Within the Department of Defense and a Plan to Expand Availability,* the DoD set a goal of meeting 80 percent of the potential need for child care among military families. In recent years, targets have been expressed in numbers of spaces. The current goal is to provide 215,412 spaces by fiscal year 2007.

To evaluate progress toward that goal, DoD needs information on the magnitude of that potential need. For a number of years, the DoD has been using a formula that translates the basic demographic characteristics of the military population into child care need as a tool to get this information. The Office of the Secretary of Defense (OSD) asked the RAND Corporation to collect data on child care need and child care choices, assess the validity of the DoD formula, and recommend improvements to the formula. Data for the assessment came from a survey of military families about child care issues, conducted in 2004.

This technical report describes and analyzes the results of that survey. It documents survey methods, defines three outcomes of potential interest to DoD (reported child-care usage, unmet child-care need, and unmet child-care preference), presents detailed results of an analysis of these outcomes among military families, and analyzes the relationship between these outcomes and characteristics of military families and military installations. A companion RAND monograph applies the results of the analyses reported here to address the validity of the Department of Defense child-care-demand formula (Moini, Zellman, and Gates, 2006).

This report will be of interest to officials responsible for DoD child-care policy and other quality of life issues. It should also be of interest to child care managers in other federal organizations, child care researchers, and child care policymakers at the national, state, and local levels who grapple with the issue of estimating the need for child care.

This report is part of a series of RAND reports on military child care:

- *Improving the Delivery of Military Child Care: An Analysis of Current Operations and New Approaches* (R-4145, 1992) examined military child-care operations prior to the implementation of the Military Child Care Act (MCCA) of 1989.

- *Examining the Effects of Accreditation on Military Child Development Center Operations and Outcomes* (MR-524, 1994) analyzed a key aspect of the MCCA: accreditation of centers.
- *Examining the Implementation and Outcomes of the Military Child Care Act of 1989* (MR-665, 1998) analyzed the many changes that the MCCA brought about.
- *Examining the Cost of Military Child Care* (MR-1415, 2002) determined the cost of providing care in military child development centers and homes.

This research was conducted for the Department of Defense Office of Family Policy within the Forces and Resources Policy Center of the RAND National Defense Research Institute (NDRI). NDRI, a division of the RAND Corporation, is a federally funded research and development center sponsored by the Office of the Secretary of Defense, the Joint Staff, the unified commands, and the defense agencies.

Reader comments should be sent to the authors at RAND, P.O. Box 2138, Santa Monica, CA 90407-2138, or Susan_Gates@rand.org. For more information on RAND's Forces and Resources Policy Center, contact the Director, James Hosek. He can be reached by email at James_Hosek@rand.org; by phone at 310-393-9411, extension 7138; or by mail at the RAND Corporation, 1776 Main Street, Santa Monica, California 90407-2138. More information about RAND is available at http://www.rand.org.

Contents

Tables

Summary

The military child-care system has received nationwide recognition for providing high-quality child care to a large number of military families (Campbell et al., 2000). The military provides care for as long as 12 hours per day in child development centers (CDCs), and even longer if necessary in family child care (FCC) homes.[1] However, in spite of the vast size of the system, access to child care is far from universal within the Department of Defense (DoD). Many families remain on waiting lists for military child care or seek out alternatives off base.

DoD is committed to meeting the child care need among military families. To monitor progress toward that goal, DoD requires a meaningful measure of that need. The purpose of this report is to improve understanding of the child care choices that military families make and the factors that might influence those choices, and to assess the extent to which DoD is meeting the child care needs of military families. This report will assist DoD in assessing the effectiveness of the current DoD child-care-demand formula, which translates the basic demographic characteristics of the military population into child care need as a tool to get information on the magnitude of the potential need.

This Report Estimates the Factors Influencing the Use of and the Unmet Need for Child Care Among Military Families

This report documents the results of a survey of 1,137 active-duty military families, including activated Reservists, regarding child care use. We analyze these survey data to estimate the relationship between individual family characteristics and installation characteristics and the probability that the family uses any nonparental child care, uses DoD-sponsored child care, has unmet need for child care, and has undermet need for child care. Through this analysis, we develop a richer understanding of the extent to which DoD is meeting the need for child care among military families. This empirically based understanding provides the basis for an assessment of the DoD child-care-demand formula provided in a related RAND report (Moini, Zellman, and Gates, 2006).

As an employer of many individuals with dependent children, DoD is concerned that parents who need some form of child care in order to work receive that care. It is also concerned that the quality of the care received is high enough that parents do not worry about their children and can focus their attention on their work. The basic questions are whether

---

[1] The services use different terms to describe FCC, including child development homes.

military parents are able to access some type of formal child care when they want it and to what extent they are satisfied with the care they are using.

There are a number of ways to think about and measure the concepts that lead to preference for and use of care. In this report, we avoid use of the term "child care demand." *Demand* is a technical economic term that relates the price charged by suppliers for a specific good or service to the amount of a product or service desired by consumers. In this report, then, we avoid focusing on demand, because the word *demand* can be interpreted in a manner that is inconsistent with its technical meaning. Instead, we consider both the use of formal child care and the extent to which parental needs are being met. We relate these "outcomes" to observable information about military families and the communities in which they live.

In approaching the issue of *need,* we articulate definitions for four key outcomes of potential interest to DoD. First, we consider parents who report that they would like to use a formal child-care arrangement but are not currently doing so. We define such parents as expressing *unmet need.* This group may include parents who care for their children themselves, as well as parents who rely on friends, older siblings, or other relatives. We also consider an alternative issue that is related to unmet need: Parents who report that they are likely or very likely to leave the military because of child care issues. Some of these families may be "served" by the system in the sense that they have an arrangement (even a DoD-sponsored arrangement) that they use. However, these parents expressed in the survey that some aspects of their child care arrangements are inadequate to the point that they may leave the military. We also consider *unmet preference,* which describes families who report using some form of care that is not their first choice. An understanding of unmet preference may help DoD consider the range of policy tools that could be used to better meet the needs of military families. Finally, we conduct an empirical analysis of the child care choices that families make.

Findings

Our findings are based on information gathered through a survey of military families with dependent children between the ages of 0 and 12 years. The survey, which covers a wide range of child care issues, was fielded between February and August 2004. The survey response rate was low (34 percent) but typical of recent surveys of military personnel. In interpreting the findings, readers should keep in mind the low response rate and the fact that response rates differed by the service, rank, race, and gender of the military member selected. In reporting the findings, we weight survey responses to correct for such observable nonresponse bias.

Unmet Need

Nearly 9 percent of parents responding to the survey reported having unmet need, defined by indicating that they would like to use a formal child-care arrangement but are not currently doing so. Parents of pre–school-aged children are neither more nor less likely than parents of school-aged children to express unmet need.

Among parents of children aged 0 to 5 years, dual-military families are the least likely to report unmet need, whereas families with civilian nonworking spouses are most likely to report unmet need (about 19 percent). The analysis also suggests that the income level of the military family affects the likelihood of unmet need. Compared with families that had earnings greater than $75,000 in 2003, those earning less than $50,000 per year were more likely to report unmet need. Families on the low end of the income distribution that express unmet need may be in a situation in which a lack of child care availability is preventing a civilian spouse from working outside the home.

Among families of children between the ages of 6 and 12 years, we found no relationship between family or installation characteristics and reports of unmet need.

Unmet Preference

While relatively few families reported unmet child-care need, many more reported unmet preference. Of survey respondents, 22 percent reported that their current child-care arrangement is not their first choice. Parents of pre–school-aged children are more likely to report unmet preference (30 percent) than are parents of school-aged children (19 percent).

Among parents of pre–school-aged children, those families with military members whose work hours vary are more likely to report unmet preference, which suggests that existing child-care arrangements may not match well with irregular military schedules. Relative to Air Force families, Army and Marine Corps families are less likely to report unmet child-care preference.

Among parents of school-aged children, we found that those using civilian-run formal child-care arrangements were more likely than those using DoD-sponsored arrangements or parental care to report unmet preference. Dual-military families with school-aged children were also more likely to report unmet preference than were single parents of school-aged children. Finally, families who have variable work hours were more likely to report unmet preference.

Approximately one-third of families that expressed unmet preference stated that their preferred option is DoD-sponsored care. This response is particularly true for parents of pre–school-aged children. Fifty-one percent of parents of pre–school-aged children who expressed unmet preference state a preference for DoD CDC care. However, preference for DoD-sponsored care is not universal. Many families who currently use DoD-sponsored care state a preference for some other form of care. Among parents of pre–school-aged children, we found no statistically significant relationship between the type of care currently used and the likelihood of expressing unmet preference, suggesting that families using DoD-sponsored care are no more (or less) likely to be dissatisfied with their current arrangements than are other families. Among parents of school-aged children, we found that parents using civilian-run formal child-care arrangements are twice as likely to express unmet preference, compared with parents using any other option.

Likelihood of Leaving the Military

Given that few families reported unmet child-care need, it is somewhat surprising that 21 percent of families responding to our survey reported that it was likely or very likely that they would leave the military because of child care issues. Families with pre–school-aged children were much more likely to report a propensity to leave the military (36 percent) than were parents of school-aged children (15 percent). Since our analysis does not control for military rank or years of service, this difference is most likely due to the fact that families with older children have more years of military service and a greater commitment to the military career.

Family status and service-related issues appear to have a strong relationship with plans to leave the service. Among families, with a pre–school-aged child, we found that dual-military families report a higher propensity to leave the military due to child care issues than single parents. Among families with school-aged children, families with a working civilian spouse are less likely than single parents to report such a propensity.

The type of child care arrangement currently used also relates to reports of the likelihood of leaving the service. Compared with families using the DoD CDC, families using all other care arrangements, including DoD FCC, are *less* likely to report that they are considering leaving the military due to child care issues (although the difference between DoD CDC and formal civilian care is significant only at the 10-percent level.) Families of military officers are less likely to report that they have considered leaving the military due to child care issues than are families of enlisted personnel.

Among families with school-aged children, those with an employed civilian spouse are less likely to be considering leaving the military due to child care issues compared with single parents. Families living more than 20 miles from the installation are substantially more likely than families living on base to be considering leaving the military. Reservists are more likely to report having considered leaving the service.

We also found that families who express unmet preference are much more likely to say that they are likely to leave the military due to child care issues, illustrating an important link between these two outcomes.

Child Care Choice

Military families use a wide variety of child care arrangements, with parental care being the most prevalent. In modeling child care choice, we first considered the question of whether a family uses parental care or not; then, for those families who do not use parental care, we explored the question of which child care option they would choose. Not surprisingly, the factors that influence the decision to use parental care differ from the factors influencing the type of care used, and the factors differ by child age.

Decision to Use Parental Care. Compared with single military parents,[2] dual-military families are less likely to use parental care, and civilian families with nonworking spouses are more likely to use parental care. Families who live off base, but within 10 miles of the installation, are more likely than those on base to use parental care.

Among families with pre–school-aged children, we also found that families with a civilian working spouse are more likely to use parental care. Families who live in a community with a greater supply of child care workers are less likely to use parental care for their pre–school-aged children. This finding is consistent with our hypothesis that, in areas in which the supply of non-DoD child-care options is greater, civilian spouses are more likely to work outside the home and to use that care.

Among families of school-aged children, we found that families with incomes less than $50,000 per year are more likely than families with incomes of more than $75,000 per year to use parental care. Families whose highest-ranking military member is an officer are more likely than families of enlisted personnel to use parental care for their school-aged chil-

---

[2] Although it appears counterintuitive that single parents would use parental care, one should keep in mind that a child of a single military parent often has another parent who may be available to provide care. Our survey data reveal that all of the single parents who report using parental care are male military members who use care by the mother.

dren. Compared with Air Force families, Army and Marine Corps families are more likely to use parental care for their school-aged children. Finally, families living in areas with higher median incomes are more likely to use parental care for their school-aged children.

Choice Among Nonparental Care Options. Among families with pre–school-aged children, we considered the choice among four options: DoD CDC care, DoD FCC, formal civilian child care, and other care. The "other" category includes nanny care, relative care, or informal child-care options. The first thing we noted is that family income plays a significant role in child care choice.[3] Families earning less than $75,000 per year are less likely to use FCC than are families earning more than $75,000 per year. We also found that families whose work hours vary are less likely to use FCC.

Proximity to the installation is also an important factor in child care choice. Families living between 11 and 20 miles from the installation are less likely to use FCC than are families that live on base. Across the board, families living off base are more likely to use formal civilian child-care options, and the propensity to use civilian child care increases as the distance from the installation increases. Families who live off base but near the installation are more likely to use other care options. Relative to the Air Force, survey respondents in the Marine Corps were less likely to choose FCC or formal civilian-care options. Reservists were more likely to use FCC and other care options over the CDC. Families living in areas with higher median incomes are less likely to use formal civilian-care options, whereas families living in areas with a high supply of child care workers are more likely to use civilian, formal care options and other, informal care options as opposed to the CDC.

When we examined child care choice for families with school-aged children, we considered three options: DoD-sponsored care (including DoD-operated youth centers, school-aged care (SAC) facilities, FCC, and CDC care),[4] formal civilian child care, and other, informal care options. Again, we found a relationship between various family and installation characteristics and child care choice.

Families who have another child between the ages of 13 and 18 years are much more likely to use other informal care options relative to those who do not. Families with a civilian spouse who does not work outside the home but who use some form of nonparental care are much less likely to use DoD-sponsored forms of care for their school-aged children than are single military parents. Across the board, families living off base are more likely to use formal civilian child-care options and other informal options over the DoD-sponsored child-care options. Families who live in areas in which the female unemployment rate is high are more likely to use other, informal types of child care. Families of officers are more likely to use formal civilian-care options and informal care options, relative to families of enlisted members.

Child Care and Military Readiness

Child care issues do appear to influence the readiness of military members, and the effect appears to be greater for female military members than for males. Among families with a military father, 22 percent of survey respondents reported that the military father was late to work due to child care issues in the past month. For families with a military mother, 51 per-

---

[3] Comparisons discussed in this paragraph are relative to the probability of using DoD CDC care.

[4] Although some CDCs provide care for school-aged children, most CDCs focus on providing care for pre–school-aged children.

cent reported that the military mother was late to work due to child care issues in the past month. Forty-seven percent of families with a civilian spouse reported that the spouse was late to work due to child care issues during the past month.

Parents also miss work due to child care issues (i.e., when the child care provider is unavailable or the child is sick and cannot attend). Among families with a military father, 7 percent of survey respondents reported that the military father missed work due to child care issues in the past month. For military mothers, the figure was 37 percent. For families with a civilian spouse, the figure was 21 percent for the civilian spouse. Clearly, female military members and civilian spouses are carrying a bigger load in terms of child care, covering for child care inadequacies more than do male military members.

Conclusions

Unmet Child Care Need Is Not Prevalent Among Military Families

Just under 10 percent of military families reported unmet child-care need. While this percentage is low, DoD may be concerned that it is not zero. We found that unmet need is much more prevalent among families with pre–school-aged rather than school-aged children. Families with a civilian working spouse are more likely to express unmet need, as are families earning less than $50,000 per year. These findings suggest that policies that give dual-military and single parents a preference for DoD-sponsored care may be effective in reducing unmet need among these populations.

Unmet Preference Is More Common Than Unmet Need

A larger proportion of military families—22 percent—reported unmet preference for child care. Again, we found a greater prevalence of unmet preference among families with pre–school-aged children. Families had unmet preference for different types of care. Overall, 49 percent of the families who reported unmet preference stated that their preferred form of care is one that is provided by DoD. This finding suggests that DoD may need to use a wide variety of policy tools if it is to better meet the child care "demands" of military families.

Child Care Concerns May Influence Retention Decisions

Nearly one-third of survey respondents report that it is likely or very likely that child care issues would lead them to leave the military. This response would seem to support the notion that child care is a retention issue. However, it is important to emphasize that the fact that individuals report that they are likely to leave the service does not mean that they actually act on that sentiment. Further information would be needed to determine whether individuals who express a propensity to leave the service due to child care issues actually do so.

Nevertheless, families with pre–school-aged children were much more likely to report a propensity to leave the military. This difference may be partially due to the fact that the parents of older children tend to be older themselves and to have a longer tenure in and stronger commitment to the military career.

Dual-Military and Single-Parent Families Experience Challenges

Despite the fact that DoD policy gives special priority to dual-military and single-parent families in terms of accessing DoD-sponsored child-care options, these families are much more likely to report that they plan to leave the military due to child care issues—even though these families are less likely to report unmet need.

Housing Patterns Influence Use of DoD-Sponsored Care

The distance between a family's home and the installation is strongly related to the type of child care it uses. Families that live off base are less likely to use DoD-sponsored child-care options, and the propensity to use DoD-sponsored care is lower for families that live farther from base. It appears that many families that live off base do not find DoD-sponsored care, which is typically located on the installation, to be a convenient option. These families do seem to find other options that meet their needs.

It may be that while DoD-sponsored care is able to meet the needs of many, if not most, families who live on base, those families have few other options if they cannot be accommodated by DoD-sponsored care. This fact suggests that the housing patterns of military families stationed on a particular installation are an important characteristic for DoD to consider in deciding how to allocate its child care resources.

DoD CDC Users Appear to Have a Weaker Attachment to the Military

The conventional wisdom is that DoD CDC care is the most sought-after and convenient type of child care among military families. Certainly, waiting lists are long, and the subsidy provided to families who use this type of care is larger than the subsidy available for any other type of care. It is therefore surprising that our analysis reveals that families who use the DoD CDCs are more likely than families who use other care options to report that they are likely to leave the military due to child care issues. Given that the DoD heavily subsidizes care provided in the CDCs, and provides little or no subsidy for other options, DoD may be interested in more fully understanding the attitudes of CDC families.

Local Market Conditions Are Related to the Child Care Choices That DoD Families Make

Although DoD-sponsored care is an important option for military families, it is not the only option. Our analysis reveals that families with pre–school-aged children who live in areas with lower median incomes are more likely to use civilian sponsored care, and families who live in areas with a greater supply of child care workers are more likely to use other child care.

The relationship between median income and use of civilian-sponsored child care may reflect the implications of differences in cost of living. Since the income of military families does not vary much by locale, military families who live in affluent communities may be less willing to pay the market price for civilian child care than military families who live in poorer communities. Therefore, characteristics of the local community may be important determinants of the relative need for DoD-sponsored care. Attention to these conditions may help DoD to more effectively allocate its child care resources.

Results from This Study May Help Inform DoD Policy Decisions Related to Child Care

In a companion report (Moini, Zellman and Gates, 2006), we apply the results of this study to the question of how DoD characterizes and responds to child care need. That report recommends that DoD consider a broader range of child care outcomes and clearly articulate those that are most important in developing child care policies. We recommend that DoD consider the factors that influence child care outcomes in designing policy responses, and we suggest that DoD consider additional options to address child care need. Such options might include child care vouchers, subsidized spaces in civilian centers, subsidized wraparound care,[5] or support for after-school programs in the community.

DoD recently introduced a new program called "Operation: Military Child Care" that can serve as an example of a type of policy option DoD might want to pursue further. The program helps active-duty, Reserve, and National Guard families who do not have access to DoD-sponsored care on base to find child care, and will defray the cost of that care while military members of these families are mobilized or deployed. Clear DoD guidance, combined with a package of options that extend beyond creating spaces in DoD-sponsored care, holds promise of better utilizing child care resources to promote DoD goals and promote family choice and child well-being.

---

[5] *Wraparound care* is child care that is provided before a CDC or FCC opens and after it closes. CDCs and FCCs typically have standard hours of operation, but military families often have workdays (or have to pull 24-hour shifts) that extend beyond the hours of operation.

Acknowledgments

We thank all of the military families who took the time to fill out the Military Child Care Survey or participate in our focus groups. This research would not have been possible without their input.

We are indebted to our sponsors, Jan Witte and Barbara Thomson of the Office of Children and Youth in the Department of Defense. We appreciate their support in all aspects of the project, and their valuable feedback and guidance.

Scott Seggerman and Kit Tong of the Defense Manpower Data Center (DMDC) provided us with access to data on military families with dependent children and drew the survey sample for us. Our complicated sample design required much hard work on their part, and we are indebted to them for that effort.

We thank our RAND colleague Jennifer Hawes-Dawson, who effectively managed the fielding of the survey; Jon Scott, who cleaned the data and set up the data files; and Claude Messan Setodji, who consulted with us on survey sample selection and weighting issues. Jennifer Kavanagh recoded some of the variables after the survey was completed.

Charles Baum and Ashlesha Datar provided useful comments on an earlier draft.

Donna White and Christopher Dirks provided helpful secretarial support. Kristin Leuschner helped revise sections of the document to improve clarity. Marian Branch carefully edited the final copy.

Acronyms

AGI	adjusted gross income
APF	appropriated fund
BAH	Basic Allowance for Housing
CCDBG	Child Care and Development Block Grant
CDC	child development center
CDF	Children's Defense Fund
CDP	Child Development Program
CDS	Child Development Services
COLA	cost of living allowance
DEERS	Defense Enrollment Eligibility Reporting System
DHHS	U.S. Department of Health and Human Services
DLA	Defense Logistics Agency
DMDC	Defense Manpower Data Center
DoD	Department of Defense
DoDI	Department of Defense Instruction
FCC	family child care
FTE	full-time equivalent
FY	fiscal year
GAO	Government Accountability Office
GIS	geographic information systems
GS	government service
GSA	General Services Administration
IIA	independence of irrelevant alternatives
MCCA	Military Child Care Act of 1989
NAEYC	National Association for the Education of Young Children
NAFCC	National Association of Family Child Care
NSACA	National School-Age Child Alliance
PCS	Permanent Change of Station

| SAC | school-aged care |
| TANF | Temporary Assistance to Needy Families |

CHAPTER ONE

Introduction

In recent years, much has been written about whether the supply of child care in this country is adequate to meet the demand among working families, particularly families of low- and middle-income levels. This question is of particular importance to the Department of Defense (DoD), the largest supplier of employer-sponsored child care in the country. According to the Government Accountability Office (GAO, 1989), DoD considers child care availability and quality to be readiness issues. Lack of child care creates conflicts between parental and mission responsibilities: If parents have no child care, they may need to miss duty time in order to care for their children. If parents are forced to make informal child-care arrangements, they may perceive this care to be of low quality and may be distracted from duty as they worry about their children's welfare. Such distractions also degrade readiness.

The large scale of military child care reflects an enormous workforce and unique child-care needs. It is understood, for example, that the frequent Permanent Change of Station (PCS) moves that personnel must make reduce the likelihood that military families can rely on extended family members for child care. Work hours that may extend well beyond the normal workday also present a challenge. Training exercises that may require military members to report for duty at unusual hours and/or for extended periods also complicate child care need. Dual military families in particular may need care at nonstandard times.

In recent years, the DoD has set percentage targets for meeting some share of the potential need for child care among military families.[1] More recently, the DoD has set targets in terms of numbers of spaces—that is, gross capacity, or total number of children that can be served at any one time.[2] The current goal is to provide 215,412 spaces by fiscal year 2007. Currently, the DoD provides approximately 176,000 spaces (http://www.mfrc-dodqol.org/MCY/mm_cdc.htm).

To estimate the magnitude of child care need among military service personnel, the DoD uses a formula incorporating installation-level and other demographic data, including "a combination of national and military statistical trends to determine the number of potential child care users."[3] These data include number of single parents with children under 12 years of age living with them, number of dual military families, number of families with mothers working outside the home full-time and part-time, and number of DoD civilians working on the installation.

---

[1] For example, in 1992, the goal was to meet 80 percent of the potential need.

[2] This gross capacity measure does not reflect the age of children served or other aspects of the care provided.

[3] Letter to Honorable Les Aspin, Chairman, Committee on Armed Forces, House of Representatives, December 31, 1990, from Christopher Jehnn, Assistant Secretary of Defense (Force Management and Personnel).

Because the formula is based solely on demographic data, DoD was concerned that the formula might not be addressing all relevant aspects of child care need. OSD asked the RAND Corporation to assess the validity of its demand formula and to recommend improvements. As an initial step in this process, RAND conducted focus groups on eight installations. On the basis of those focus groups, RAND developed a survey designed to better understand parental preferences and other factors that may affect child care need. This report summarizes the results of that survey and an analysis of survey data. A related RAND report (Moini, Zellman, and Gates, 2006) draws on this information to evaluate the DoD's child-care-demand formula.

The Military Child-Care System

Military child care is provided as part of a system of care designed to meet the needs of military families as children age, so that children can be served by the DoD child-care system from age six weeks until age 12 years. A range of different settings enables the system to meet parents' needs for reliable, high-quality care while recognizing parental preferences concerning environment, size (number of children cared for in that provider setting), and flexibility. The military provides care for as much as 12 hours a day in child development centers (CDCs), and even longer if necessary in family child care (FCC) homes.[4] For those families with more limited need, care may also be provided on a part-time and an hourly basis in CDCs and FCCs in many locations. Before- and after-school programs are available to care for school-aged children in a center-like setting; youth programs provide a relatively unstructured but supervised setting for older school-aged children.

Child care is costly to provide, and the military child-care system requires careful planning. For example, CDCs must be requested years in advance to allow adequate time for such planning and for construction. Child development centers' construction projects must compete with other projects that some may view as more urgent.

The System Provides Significant Subsidies for CDC Use
Within the military child-care system, different types of care are subsidized at dramatically different rates (see Zellman and Gates, 2002). The term *subsidy* has different meanings for different types of care. For CDC care, it reflects the difference between the cost to DoD of providing the care and the price charged to parents. It is important to note that, for military child care, the subsidy is usually not visible to parents; although weekly CDC fees are well below market rates, parents may not be aware of the substantially higher fees in the civilian sector.

For FCC care, the subsidy reflects a payment from DoD to FCC providers that often covers only insurance or other incidentals, or is designed to promote a DoD goal, such as increased infant care. This payment, which supplements parent fees, is not typically visible to

---

[4] FCC is child care provided in a person's home. A CDC is a dedicated child-care facility. These are generic terms that apply to child care in the general community and in the DoD system. All U.S. states license child care providers (both CDCs and FCCs). DoD has its own approval and inspection process. A DoD FCC is an FCC that has been approved by DoD. Most installations will only approve military spouses operating an FCC in an on-base home. But, increasingly, installations are moving to approve off-base FCCs as well (usually those run by military spouses or the spouses of retired military).

parents. For civilian care, a subsidy would reflect a payment from DoD to the civilian provider to supplement parent fees. This type of subsidy would be more visible to parents, particularly if the subsidy were delivered in the form of a voucher.

In the DoD, CDC care is highly subsidized, there are only limited subsidies for FCC, and, in most cases, no subsidy is provided for non-DoD care.[5] For CDC care, the size of the subsidy depends on the difference between the cost to provide the care and the fees that parents are charged. The cost to provide care varies dramatically by the age of the child (Zellman and Gates, 2002), whereas parent fees depend on family income, not child age.[6] As a result, the size of the CDC subsidy is generally larger for families with younger children and/or lower family incomes.[7]

In contrast to the high level of CDC subsidy, there is limited subsidy assistance for military families who use FCC. Since FCC providers may set their own fees, the price charged to parents may be higher or lower than that for CDC care, depending on both fee levels and family income. In general, families with lower income face higher fees in an FCC relative to a CDC, whereas families in the highest income categories may face lower fees in an FCC than in a CDC. Some installations provide subsidies to FCC providers. Some subsidies help providers with general costs, such as insurance; most further specific DoD child-care goals, such as increased infant spaces, extended-hours care, and care for children with special needs.

When an FCC provider claims a subsidy, she must agree to limit her fees to those charged by the CDC. Such policies obviously benefit parents and remove a disincentive for lower income families to use an FCC; however, these subsidy policies are not systematic across services. Limited subsidies for FCCs have reduced their attractiveness to military parents and limited the value of FCC as part of the military child-care system. The flexibility that FCC can provide in terms of hours and days of care may be underexploited because of the high price some parents face relative to CDC care.

Similarly, with a few exceptions, no subsidies are available for military families who use civilian child care. Because the quality of child care available in the civilian market varies dramatically, it is not appropriate or informative to compare the average cost of DoD care with the average cost of civilian care. Over 95 percent of DoD CDCs are accredited,[8]

---

[5] These differences are largely driven by the provisions of the Military Child Care Act of 1989 (MCCA). The intent of the MCCA was to improve the quality, availability, and affordability of child care across military installations. The key lever for ensuring affordability was to require that each dollar spent by parents in CDC fees be matched by a dollar of appropriated funds (taxpayer dollars). CDC fees were to be based on total family income, for which families were organized into five fee categories.

[6] DoD established a fee schedule that defined a range of acceptable fees that may be charged by DoD CDCs. Families were divided into five income categories, and fees varied by category. For the 2004–2005 school year, allowable parent fees under the DoD fee schedule ranged from a minimum of $43 per week for families with incomes below $28,000 per year to a maximum of $126 per week for families with incomes over $70,000 per year. Installations in high-cost-of-living areas are allowed to set slightly higher fees.

[7] For example, Zellman and Gates (2002) estimated that it cost DoD approximately $12,000 per year to provide infant care in CDCs in 1998. Parent fees for the middle-income category covered 27 percent of that cost. It cost DoD about $6,600 to provide pre–school-aged care, and parent fees for the middle-income category covered 53 percent of that cost. The largest subsidy is provided to parents of infants in low-income categories; the smallest subsidy goes to parents of older children in the highest-income category.

[8] Accreditation by the National Association for the Education of Young Children (NAEYC) is a voluntary process that holds centers to a higher quality standard than state licensing. To become accredited, a center must engage in a three-step process that includes self-study, a site-validation visit, and a commission decision. The process must be repeated every three years. An accreditation process is available for family-based care through the National Association of Family Child Care

whereas the rate of accreditation in the civilian sector is only 8 percent (Campbell et al., 2000). Therefore, while it is likely that some of the civilian child-care options available to military families are less expensive than the CDC, other *accredited* options are substantially more expensive if they are available at all.[9]

Parents also expressed strong preferences for CDC care (Macro International, 1999; Zellman et al., 1992). Military families who preferred CDCs cited issues of cost, convenience, reliability, and safety (see Appendix A for results from focus groups with military parents).[10] Some of that preference can be attributed to the attractive CDCs that have been built in recent years; part of that preference is based on parental concerns about isolation and lack of oversight in FCCs; and, part of that preference is attributable to the lower level of dependability that an individual (as compared to an institution) can provide. But some part can also be explained by the fact that, for parents in the lower fee categories, this inherently less-attractive child-care alternative also costs them more when no subsidy is provided by DoD. As a result of these price differences, there are waiting lists for DoD CDC care on nearly all DoD installations with a CDC.[11]

The System Provides Special Preference for Dual-Military and Single-Parent Families

DoD policy stipulates that the child care system should give priority to single parents and dual-military parents.[12] In practice, many installations accomplish this objective by managing their CDC waitlists in such a way that priority is given to single parents and dual-military families. Military families that include a civilian spouse who neither works outside the home nor is a student are generally not eligible for CDC care. CDC waiting lists generally include high numbers of children from the youngest age groups (Zellman and Gates, 2002), but the system's capacity to care for younger children (infants and pre-toddlers) is lower than that for older children (pre–school-aged children). The relativity small capacity of CDCs to serve the youngest children reflects the reality of a fee policy based on family income and the fact that the cost of providing care is highest for the youngest children.

To ensure adequate funding, DoD CDCs typically have far more spaces for pre–school-aged children than for infants. As a result, waiting lists are very long for the youngest children, but may be nonexistent for pre–school-aged children; often, such spaces go begging because care for four- or five-year-olds can be purchased more cheaply in the community.

(NAFCC) and, for school-aged care, through the National School-Age Care Alliance (NSACA). See NAEYC (1991) for more detail on the accreditation process.

[9] All states require child care providers (either CDCs or FCCs) to be licensed. It is technically illegal to operate unlicensed child care. States have different requirements, but they look at staff-to-child ratios, safety issues, health practices, etc. Accreditation is a voluntary process that sets higher quality standards. Zellman and Gates (2002) reported that accredited centers that are subsidized by civilian employers charge fees that are substantially higher than those charged by military child-care centers. Accredited centers that are not subsidized would presumably charge even higher fees.

[10] Although, in general, military parents express preferences for CDC care, some CDC users are critical of some aspects of the CDCs, such as the fee schedule, hours of operation, and policies related to administering medicines.

[11] Office of Family Policy, U.S. Department of Defense, "Need for Child Care Spaces by Service" (March 2000).

[12] Department of Defense Instruction 6060.2, "Child Development Programs," January 19, 1993.

Objectives

The purpose of the overall study is to assess the accuracy and effectiveness of current approaches to estimating the need for child care among military families.[13] The purpose of this technical report is to provide an empirically based description of child care need among military families and an analysis of the relationship between need, family characteristics, and characteristics of the locale. In this report, we propose four concrete outcomes that are indicative of child care need: unmet need, unmet preference, propensity to leave the military due to child care issues, and type of child care used. We then analyze the relationship among these outcomes and family characteristics and community characteristics. A companion report applies the results of this analysis to examine the DoD's child-care-demand formula (Moini, Zellman, and Gates, 2006).

Data

Our analyses are based on information gathered through a survey, fielded between February and August 2004, of military families with dependent children between the ages of 0 and 12 years. The sample, which was drawn by the Defense Manpower Data Center (DMDC) from Defense Enrollment Eligibility Reporting System (DEERS) data, included families of active-duty military members, including activated Reservists, stationed in the United States. Although being stationed in the United States was a criterion for being included in the survey sample, the military member may have been deployed abroad at the time of the survey. Surveys were sent to home mailing addresses and could be completed by a military parent or a civilian spouse.

The survey covers a wide range of issues related to child care demand. The survey asks individuals to report their current child-care arrangements for one particular randomly chosen child in the family. The survey asks about the primary child-care arrangement and the reasons for that choice. The survey also asks families to report any additional child-care arrangements used for that child and the reasons for selecting those arrangements. The survey asks questions about the relationship between child care on the one hand and military readiness and retention on the other. There are questions about the most recent deployment of a military member and how that influenced the need for child care. The survey also asks about family characteristics so that we might understand how those characteristics influence child care choices and career choices.

---

[13] Although waiting lists for child care spaces provide a potential source of information on child care need, it is widely recognized that they are an imperfect measure of the need for child care. In 1992, DoD established a requirement for installations to maintain different waiting lists for DoD-provided care. There is a list for families with *unmet need*, which is defined for the purposes of the waiting list as those in which a parent cannot work because of lack of care or those that are using unsatisfactory care that is costly (determined as 20 percent more than the highest DoD fee category) or that is unlicensed. There is another list for families with *unmet preference*, or those with their child in a satisfactory child-care arrangement but who wish to have them in another kind of care. Parents may be reluctant to place their children on certain waiting lists because the waiting lists are too long. Conversely, people may remain on a list even after they have found an alternative care arrangement.

The survey responses have been merged with information on the characteristics of the local community in which the military member is stationed. Specifically, we included zip-code information on unemployment rates and median income. In addition, we constructed measures of child care supply within the local area, using census data.

The survey content was informed by a series of focus groups with military parents. We conducted 21 focus groups at 8 installations across the country from November 2002 through July 2003. We visited two installations from each service. Focus group participants included mothers and fathers. In most cases, the participating parent was a military member. Participants represented single-parent and dual-military families, as well as families with a civilian spouse. In addition to the focus groups, we conducted interviews with the directors of child and youth services and the directors of resource and referral and/or family child care at each installation to get an overview of CDC and FCC availability, impressions of child care demand, off-base options for child care, and the programs and policies in place to meet the particular needs of families on the installation. These focus groups are summarized in Appendix A.

The Demand for Military Child Care Is an Illusive Concept

To the extent possible, we avoid use of the term *child care demand* in this report. Because the term is often used in discussing the amount of child care that DoD should be providing, we explain why we are not talking about child care demand below.

Demand is a technical economic term that has specific connotations that do not apply to this study; indeed, the term is often not applicable in the many discussions in which it is used. *Demand* relates the price charged by suppliers for a specific good or service to the amount of a product or service desired by consumers. For most goods and services, the relationship between price and quantity demanded is assumed to be negative. In other words, holding the characteristics of the good or service, such as quality, constant, consumers will want to purchase less of it as the price goes up. It is important to note that demand is not a single number; rather, it is a functional relationship between the price and characteristics of a good or service on the one hand and the amount of that good or service that customers demand on the other hand. The amount of a good or service demanded can, and often does, change as the price or other characteristics of the good or service change.

In the case of child care, estimating a demand function is complicated by several factors. First, "child care" is not a homogenous service. Characteristics of child care arrangements vary dramatically, as do parental preferences concerning those characteristics. For example, some parents prefer the personal attention available in a family child-care environment, whereas others prefer the security and reliability of a child development center. Moreover, prices vary both across care types and within care types. Some civilian child-care centers charge modest fees, and others charge much higher fees, holding child age constant.[14] In most cases (here, the DoD centers are a significant exception), fees for care are higher for younger children. These higher fees reflect the higher costs of caring for younger children for whom staff-to-child ratios must be considerably higher.

---

[14] In most civilian centers, fees vary with child age. Fees decline as children age, because the cost of providing care declines as child-to-staff ratios increase.

Some child care spaces (including DoD-sponsored CDC care and some FCC, as discussed above) are subsidized, which means that the price that parents pay is lower than the actual cost of providing that care. The relationship between the amount of a service demanded and price is usually negative. If the price goes down, we expect that people will either consume more of the service or will select a higher-quality option. We expect that parents will want to purchase more care at the subsidized price than they would want (or be able) to purchase at the unsubsidized price. What this means is that when considering demand for DoD child care, subsidies change the dynamic and make it much more difficult to understand and discuss demand.

Many studies have attempted to estimate relationships among the price of care, quality of care, and the amount of care purchased in the child care market. These studies, which have focused on child care in general rather than the military child-care system, have generated some general conclusions. In a summary of the research in this area, Blau (2001, p. 83) reports that "a decrease in the price of child care increases the quantity of child care demanded and the employment rate of mothers, but does not increase the quality of care demanded." Overall, the research suggests a strong relationship between price and family income on the one hand and the amount of care demanded on the other, but a very weak relationship between price and income and child care quality.

Blau (2001) posits several reasons for the lack of a relationship between price, ability to pay, and quality. It is possible that parents simply do not value quality or consider quality to be secondary to other considerations, such as convenience and cost. Indeed, some research (e.g., Johansen, Leibowitz, and Waite, 1997) finds that location and price are the key characteristics that parents report they consider in choosing child care. Another possibility is that parents may not be capable of distinguishing between high- and low-quality care. Indeed, some argue that parents may mistakenly use fees as an indicator of quality because they do not know how to make an independent assessment. A number of organizations (e.g., Qualistar Early Learning) have been established with the mission of developing a rating system for child care providers that will make quality transparent and enable parents to fully include quality in the decisions they make about child care providers. Finally, it may be that parents do not value the same "quality" characteristics that researchers value. This last hypothesis is one put forward by Kisker and Maynard (1991). The measures of quality that researchers use to assess the quality of a child care arrangement, such as the education or training level of providers, characteristics of the curriculum used by caregivers, and the number of caregivers per child, may be less important to parents than are other aspects of the care arrangement, such as how well the child likes the caregiver. In other words, there may be a strong relationship between parents' willingness to pay for quality, but researchers do not fully understand how parents are defining *quality*.

We believe that the DoD would not find it sufficiently valuable to invest in the ongoing data collection required to assess and understand the complicated relationships that define the demand for child care. The DoD cannot gain access on a regular enough basis to detailed information on all the factors that go into a family's child care decisions to assess demand. Moreover, it would be prohibitive to keep track of all the options available to each family. Both of these kinds of data are necessary to conduct sophisticated and accurate analyses of child care demand.

However, as an employer of many individuals with dependent children who may have lost desirable child-care options because of work-related moves, DoD has shown admirable concern about child care need. More than most U.S. employers, the DoD has made notable efforts to see that parents who need some form of child care in order to show up for work every day receive that care and that the quality of the care received is high enough that parents do not worry about their children and can focus their attention on their work. The basic questions, then, for DoD are whether military parents are able to access some form of formal child care when they want it and to what extent they are satisfied with the care they are using.

In this report, then, we consider both the use of formal child care and the extent to which parental needs are being met. We relate these "outcomes" to observable information about military families and the communities in which they live.

Definitions

There are a number of ways to think about and measure the extent to which DoD is meeting the child care needs of military families. In this section, we define the key outcomes that we use in our analysis. Each of the measures provides a different perspective on the need for child care and the role of DoD in meeting that need. In selecting concepts for analysis, we focus on outcomes of potential interest to DoD. Our companion report (Moini, Zellman, and Gates, 2006) discusses the relationship between these measures and current DoD policy, as well as policy issues that would arise were DoD to focus attention on one or more of these measures.

In defining these terms, and characterizing families as having unmet need, we make a distinction between families who use formal child-care arrangements and those who use an informal arrangement. We consider an arrangement to be a *formal arrangement* if it involves providers other than friends or family members and occurs on a regular basis during working hours. Formal child-care arrangements for military families may include DoD-sponsored child development centers or family child care (FCC) homes, as well as the full range of options available to nonmilitary parents, including off-base centers, civilian FCC, and nannies. *Informal arrangements* include care provided by siblings, relatives or friends, and the child himself.[15] Parental care is a third option that falls into neither category.

We recognize that not all families want to use formal child-care arrangements. Indeed, some parents make significant sacrifices, such as requesting work on alternate shifts, to ensure that they can care for their children themselves, even if each parent works full-time. Another important category of nonusers of child care includes parents who are able to support one parent staying at home, either to exclusively care for children or to combine work at home with child care.

Unmet Need for Care

Instead of demand, we have focused attention in our analyses on *unmet need* for care. This concept can be more clearly defined and is not as seriously influenced by the issues inherent

---

[15] DoD regulations prohibit self-care by children 12 years and under. However, we asked about such care in the families we surveyed (all of whom had a child 12 and under) because we believed that self-care does occur among younger children, and we needed to understand its frequency and the circumstances under which it occurs. Assurances of confidentiality were offered to parents to encourage them to reveal such arrangements.

in using the concept of demand.[16] In defining and analyzing unmet need, we consider parents' perspective and define unmet need to exist when they report that they would like to use a formal child-care arrangement but are not currently doing so. This group may include parents who care for their children themselves, as well as parents who rely on friends, older siblings, or other relatives.

One might view our definition of *unmet need* as excessively broad. In fact, we considered several possible definitions of *unmet need*, including a focus on families who report that a lack of child care options prevents a parent from working outside the home. As it turns out, only a small fraction (2 percent) of the survey respondents fit that more-restrictive category of unmet need. This situation may be due, in part, to the fact that employment options for civilian spouses are so limited in some areas (59 percent of families with a civilian spouse report that employment options in the local area are limited or very limited) that families do not view access to child care as the primary constraint on employment.

One might also view our definition of unmet need as excessively narrow in the sense that it does not capture families who are using formal child care that is insufficient in some way. We attempt to address the issue of insufficient care through a consideration of unmet preference.

Likelihood of Leaving the Military

We also considered an alternative issue that is related to unmet need—parents who report that they are likely or very likely to leave the military because of child care issues. Note that some of these families may be "served" by the system in the sense that they have an arrangement (even a DoD-sponsored arrangement) that they use. However, these parents expressed in the survey that some aspects of their child care arrangements are inadequate to the point of propelling them to leave the military. This definition of *unmet need* may be of particular interest to the DoD.

Unmet Preference

In addition to unmet need and propensity to leave the military, we also considered the notion of *unmet preference*, which describes families who report using some form of care that is not their first choice.[17] Unmet preference is important in considering child care choices made by military parents. It may reflect a lack of availability of DoD-sponsored care for those using other forms or, conversely a lack of availability of affordable civilian-sponsored child care for those who use military child care. It may also reflect some type of inadequacy in the type of child care used.

As noted in the introduction, the military subsidizes child development centers (CDCs) quite heavily. In contrast, FCC is subsidized at a much lower level, and sometimes not at all. Other choices are not subsidized. Consequently, there may be a substantial unmet

---

[16] Still, as emphasized by Queralt and Witte (1999, p. 527), there are several ways to think about unmet need. "Operationally speaking, need or unmet need for services refers to the gap or disparity between optimal and actual levels of service provision in a geographic area." The authors note that there is no single objective measure of the "optimal" level of service. Moreover, it is possible to consider unmet need from different perspectives (e.g., a local government's, an employer's, a parent's).

[17] Unmet need is a subset of unmet preference. Any family that expresses unmet need is also characterized as having unmet preference. However, the definition of *unmet preference* also captures families that have a formal child care arrangement that they are using if it is not their first choice.

preference for CDCs. Many parents who are unable to get their children into CDCs make other arrangements that turn out to be acceptable, even desirable, over time. But strictly on monetary grounds, many parents maintain a preference for CDC care. Conversely, parents may prefer to use civilian child care (i.e., because it is more convenient to home), but that use may be precluded by the lack of subsidy for such care.

Child Care Use

We also examine child care use as an outcome of interest. Although child care use is not a measure of need, our examination of child care use allows us to describe the extent to which those who are using some form of child care are being served by the DoD system.

Scope and Limitations

This report articulates definitions of concepts that might plausibly be of interest to DoD and explores the relationships among various characteristics of military families and installations, on the one hand, and child care choice, unmet need, unmet preference, and reported likelihood of leaving the military service on the other. It does not provide an economic estimation of child care demand among military parents.

A companion to this technical report (Moini, Zellman, and Gates, 2006) applies the results of this analysis to consider policy questions related to military child care. Specifically, that report assesses the validity of the DoD child-care-demand formula as a tool for translating information on military families into measures of potential child-care need and to suggest ways that the tool might be improved, clarifies the role of the DoD formula in DoD child-care policy decisions, and discusses the factors that influence key child-care outcomes of interest to DoD.

This report documents the results of a survey conducted by RAND of active-duty military families covering child care issues. This survey was fielded from February to July 2004. Thus, responses are reflective of the period during which the DoD was engaged in a major effort in Iraq and many military members were deployed. The survey sample includes active-duty military personnel (including activated Reservists) who report having a dependent child 12 years of age or younger.

This survey focuses attention on the issues facing families stationed in the United States, because we include only individuals stationed in the United States in our survey sample. Families stationed abroad on accompanied tours face additional challenges in terms of spousal employment and access to off-base child-care options. Although stationed in the United States, the military members included in the sample may have been deployed abroad from that U.S. station. Our sample includes single parents, dual-military families, and families that include one military member who is married to a civilian.

We received a total of 1,137 responses to the survey, for a response rate of 34 percent. This response rate was disappointingly low, but typical of recent surveys of military personnel.[18] In interpreting the findings, readers should keep in mind the low response rate

---

[18] Newell et al. (2004, p. 266) document the drop in survey response rates in general, for military surveys and for U.S. Navy surveys in particular: "The Navy-wide Personnel Survey had a 52-percent response rate in 1990, a 45-percent response rate in 1996, and a 33-percent response rate in 2000." The response rate for the 2002 DoD Status of Forces survey was

and the fact that response rates differed by the service, rank, race, and gender of the military member selected. In reporting the findings and performing the analyses, we weighted survey responses to correct for observable nonresponse bias. Appendix B provides an analysis of response rates used to identify nonresponse bias. The weighting process used to correct for nonresponse bias is detailed in Chapter Three.

Organization of the Report

In Chapter Two, we provide a literature review and present some hypotheses based on that review. In Chapter Three, we present a descriptive overview of the survey, sample selection process, and our methodology for analyzing the survey results. Individuals who are not interested in this technical detail may wish to skip this chapter. Chapter Four summarizes the results of the multivariate analyses. Chapter Five provides a discussion and conclusions. Appendix A provides a summary of focus groups with military parents. Appendix B presents an analysis of survey response rates, relating them to observable characteristics of the survey sample. Appendix C contains the actual survey instrument.

---

32 percent. (Available online at http://www.defenselink.mil/releases/2003/b02252003_bt083-03.html; accessed May 10, 2005.)

CHAPTER TWO

Factors Influencing Child Care Choice and Unmet Need

There is a substantial literature on the factors expected to influence child care use and unmet need for child care services in the civilian sector. This literature suggests some relationships that we might expect to see among child care use and family and community characteristics. In general, we expected that many of the factors that influence use and need in the civilian population will also be relevant to the consideration of DoD-sponsored care. However, the military population does differ from the civilian population in significant ways. We draw on the results of focus groups that we conducted as part of this project (see Appendix A) to identify potential relationships specific to the military populations. We highlight those differences and some military-specific issues in our review of the existing literature.

Price

Prior research suggests that the price of child care is a primary factor influencing its use. Mothers are more likely to be employed outside the home, and families use more hours of child care when the price of child care is lower (Blau, 2001). The DoD child-care system provides military families with more options than those available to civilian working families. Most DoD installations operate child development centers (CDCs). The price of care in these centers is highly subsidized, especially for infants (Zellman and Gates, 2002), and the fees depend on total family income, so that families with higher incomes pay a higher weekly fee.

Unlike the situation in the civilian child-care market, DoD CDC fees vary not by child age but by family income. As discussed in Chapter One, the price of FCC is also subsidized, but in a less systematic way and to a much more limited extent. Because of the way DoD chooses to subsidize child care for military families, the relative price of DoD CDC care, DoD FCC, and off-base care varies depending on the income level of the family, the age of the child, the number of children in the family, and the location of the installation. For families with low incomes (e.g., military members of low rank) and young children, DoD CDC care is likely to be the lowest-price option. Families with higher incomes, older children, and several children are likely to find FCC or off-base care to be relatively cheaper, since off-base centers typically do not adjust fees according to parent income level, charge less for older children, and may offer discounts for the second and third child.

We therefore hypothesize that, **holding preferences constant, price factors may encourage higher-income military families more than their lower-income counterparts to use FCC or non-DoD child-care options.** Our focus groups suggested that these financial pressures may also drive **lower-income families to consider leaving the military.** However, because the quality and availability of specific care options are often correlated with price, and because preferences may not be constant across income categories, these hypothesized relationships between price and outcomes may not be observed.

Proximity

The literature suggests that most families do consider the location of a child care arrangement to be an important characteristic (Van Horn, Ramey, et al., 2001), although we are aware of no studies that have explicitly estimated parents' willingness to pay more for child care that is closer to either home or work. Our focus groups with military families suggest that they may place a greater emphasis on the proximity of the child care arrangement to work than civilian parents do because many military members need to report for duty quite early. Even if they drop the child at the child care provider right when it opens, the commute time between the child care provider and the duty location is often a factor determining whether they can report to duty on time.

Military families with an employed civilian spouse often have more flexibility, since the civilian spouse is likely to be on a different schedule from the military spouse. These families may prefer child care options that are close to home[1] or to the spouse's work location.

This distinction between the installation and home is irrelevant for families who live on base. With the exception of personnel in critical positions (such as base commander), military families can choose to live off base, and may be forced to live off base if there is a lack of on-base housing. Buddin et al. (1999) found that about half of junior and mid-grade enlisted personnel live on base and about one-third of senior enlisted personnel and officers live on base. The authors reported that most installations have a waiting list for housing. Because a member's rank and family structure determine the type of housing (e.g., size) for which they are eligible, and the supply of housing of each type is limited, excess demand for military housing exists to a similar degree at all military grades.

Our focus groups also suggested that military families may prefer on-base care, which happens to be close to the work location, for security and safety reasons. Many families view the installation as more secure than the off-base environment. On the other hand, several parents in our focus groups noted that on-base care can cause problems when base access is restricted due to high terrorist alert levels. Often, secondary caregivers are not allowed on base during these periods; the extended care the parent needs after the CDC closes becomes unavailable in such situations.

We hypothesized that, holding preference, quality, and availability constant, **single military parents and dual-military parents will be more likely than families with a civilian spouse to use on-base care,** regardless of whether or not they live on base. Similarly, **families who live on base will be more likely than families who live off base to prefer on-base care,** because it is proximate to both home and work. **Military families with a civilian spouse who works outside the home may have a greater tendency than dual-military and single-parent**

---

[1] In an analysis of employer-sponsored, on-site care, Connelly, Degraff, et al. (2001) finds that mothers who live far from the firm are less likely to use the on-site center.

families to prefer formal civilian child-care arrangements, because such care may be close to home or to the civilian spouse's work location.

Availability

Families can only use a specific child-care option if is available to them. Gordon and Chase-Lansdale (2001) found that the probability of using center-based care is higher in communities with greater center availability. In their study, in which they estimated center availability by using census data to relate the number of child care center workers to the number of children in a particular area, they found that the probability of using center care is only 15 percent in communities with 100 children per center child-care worker and 35 percent in communities with 30 children per child care center worker. Findings were similar for family day care. The authors also found that children are most likely to spend time in a child care center in metropolitan, poor zip codes and least likely to be enrolled in centers in nonmetropolitan zip codes.[2] The authors estimated a multinomial logit model with eight outcome categories that combine mother's work status and use of nonmaternal care. The model showed that the percentage of mothers employed and using center child care increases substantially when center child care becomes more available. Also, the percentage of employed mothers using no child care, father care, and family day care declines. These data suggest that centers may be the preferred form of child care among parents, and that a lack of availability rather than parental preferences may be limiting their use.

Queralt and Witte (1998) found that the supply of child care varies dramatically by census tract and that communities in socioeconomic distress have less child care available (particularly full-day center care, but also other types of formal care) than other areas. This is because parents cannot afford to pay enough to cover the costs of care.

Previous research (Zellman and Gates, 2002) suggested that the capacity of DoD CDCs to care for younger children (infants and pre-toddlers) is lower than the capacity to care for older children (pre–school-aged children). As a result, **we expected CDC care to be less available to families with younger children; therefore, we expected families to be less likely to use DoD CDC care and to be more likely to express unmet preference for this care.**

In a study of the use of on-site, employer-sponsored child care, Connelly et al. (2002) used a probit model to analyze the factors determining the use of on-site care or any center-based care. For on-site use, child age is not a significant predictor, nor is having a pre–school-aged sibling. Having a primary-school-aged sibling reduces the probability of using a center. Employees with longer job tenure are more likely to use the center, perhaps due to waitlists. Parent status as an hourly production worker, longer distance from home to factory, higher proportion of years lived in the area, and being "never married" all reduce the probability of using the center. At least some of these factors suggest that the parent cannot afford center care. A study by the National Academy of Public Administration (1997) on employer-sponsored care found that private-sector employers tend to mirror DoD in terms

---

[2] The authors used five categories to characterize the community's income and urbanicity: Metro Poor, Metro Mixed, Metro Non-poor, Nonmetro Mixed, and Nonmetro Poor. Center enrollment was low in nonmetro areas regardless of income characteristics.

of focusing attention on subsidized, on-site care, with subsidies targeted to employees with lower incomes. In contrast, child care options for federal civilian employees are rarely subsidized.

We expected the use of child care among military families to reflect similar dynamics. Because at least some military families have subsidized, employer-sponsored options available to them (either CDC or FCC care), we expected **military families to be less likely to use civilian center care, relative care, and nonrelative care outside of centers.** We also expected that **military families will be more likely to use formal civilian child care when the supply of such care in the local area is higher.**

Family Status

Our survey sample differs from traditional samples of families on child care issues because every family in our sample includes a military member. The analysis considers four distinct family types: single military parents, dual-military families, military member with a civilian working spouse, and military member with a civilian nonworking spouse. Although no literature has looked at this array of family types, we can put forward some hypotheses as to the child care choice and unmet need facing different family types, based on our focus groups and existing research on DoD child care.

On nearly all DoD installations, there are waiting lists for DoD CDC care. As described above, many installations manage their waiting lists in such a way that priority is given to single parents and dual-military families. Thus, we expected DoD CDC care to be more available to these families and **expected that unmet preference for CDC care would be greater among military families that include a civilian spouse,** and therefore are not high priority for CDC care. Military families that include a civilian spouse who neither works outside the home nor is a student are not eligible for CDC care; thus, **we expected to find some unmet preference (for DoD CDC care) among these families as well.** Some, but not all, installations also have waiting lists for DoD FCC care.

Previous research and conventional wisdom do not suggest concrete hypotheses related to the child care needs of military members married to civilian working and nonworking spouses. On the one hand, a lack of child care may prevent civilian spouses from working outside the home. These parents may have no unmet need for care, given that they are currently not working and therefore use parental care, although they would rather have formal child care and be working outside the home. We asked a question in the survey to identify families in this situation and to distinguish between families using parental care by choice rather than out of necessity from those for whom parental care represents unmet need.

Availability of Family Member to Care for Child

A nontrivial fraction of civilian families relies on relatives to care for their children while they work. The 1999 Survey of Income and Program Participation survey[3] conducted by the

---

[3] http://www.census.gov/population/www/socdemo/child/ppl-168.html.

Census Bureau indicates that 21 percent of pre–school-aged children with a working mother is cared for by a grandparent, and another 8.4 percent is cared for by another relative or sibling. For school-aged children, 19.4 percent is cared for by a grandparent and 19.9 percent by a sibling or other relative. The prevalence of relative care is higher among lower-income families and among non-white families. For some immigrant families, this source of care is highly valued, because it ensures language and cultural compatibility—something that often cannot be found in formal care settings. For many families, relative care also provides a sense of security that is perceived to be lacking when strangers care for a child.

Relative care may be paid or unpaid. Anderson and Levine (2000) found that reliance on family members to provide child care decreases as family income increases, but that low-income families are more likely to pay for the care provided by their family members. This may be a function of Temporary Assistance to Needy Families (TANF) policies that allow welfare recipients to pay family members for care that, in the absence of available government funds, they might have provided without charge. In other cases, such payment clearly substitutes for other low-income work that would be pursued if money could not be earned caring for relatives' children.

Because military families come from all across the country and have little choice concerning where they are stationed, relative care is less available to them. Indeed, one of the justifications for the establishment of the military child-care system has been the inability of military families to tap into relative care when their children are young (Zellman et al., 1992). Because of geographic separations, we **expected to observe low use of relative care among military families and some amount of unmet preference for this form of care.**

Relationship Between Child Care and Satisfaction with Military Life

Most of the literature we have reviewed examines the issue of child care use. Using data from a 1986 survey of Army families, Lakhani and Hoover (1997) explored the links among child care use, earnings, satisfaction with Army life, and retention desires of wives of U.S. Army officers. They found that child care use is sensitive to the wife's annual earnings, but not to her monthly wage,[4] and that military wives are underemployed relative to their civilian counterparts. The authors found that individuals who were dissatisfied with the cost of child care tended to be less satisfied with life in the Army in general. **Assuming that the quality of care in DoD CDCs and FCCs is equal to or higher than the quality of care in comparably priced civilian settings, we expected single parents and dual-military families to report more satisfaction with their child care options and less of a propensity to leave the military due to child care issues, because they receive preference for DoD-sponsored and subsidized child care.**

---

[4] Annual earnings are based on the number of weeks worked per year. Hosek et al. (2002) found that military spouses work fewer weeks per year than their civilian counterparts.

Summary of Hypotheses

Table 2.1 summarizes the hypotheses we have put forward in this chapter. The hypotheses posit simple relationships between individual and installation characteristics and child care outcomes. However, because of the interactions among child care preference, price, availability, and quality, individual and installation characteristics may have quite different effects on these outcomes. Our analyses will help us identify which of the relationships described by the hypotheses are supported by the empirical data.

Table 2.1
Summary of Hypotheses

Independent variable	Choice	Unmet need	Unmet preference	Leaving the military
Family status	Single military, dual military more likely to use CDC and FCC.	Greater among families with a nonworking civilian spouse	Greater unmet preference among military married to civilians.	Lower among dual-military and single-parent families.
	Families with a civilian working spouse more likely to use formal civilian care.	Lower among dual-military and single-parent families		
	Families with a non-working civilian spouse most likely to use parental care.			
Family income	Families with lower incomes are more likely to use the CDC.	Families with lower incomes are more likely to express unmet need.	Families with lower incomes are more likely to express unmet preference.	Families with lower incomes are more likely to express plans to leave the military.
Proximity to base	Families that live off base are less likely to use on-base care.	Greater among families that live off base.	Greater among families that live off base.	
Local supply of child care	Greater supply of child care in the local community will increase the use of formal civilian child care.	Greater supply of child care in the local community will decrease reports of unmet need.		

CHAPTER THREE

Methodology

In this chapter, we describe the methodology for the survey and our analysis of survey results. The complete survey instrument is included in Appendix C.

Description of Survey

The survey asked military parents about their primary and secondary child-care arrangements, and about their preferred child-care arrangement. It included questions about how cost, quality, child age, and the nature of available options, among other characteristics of care, affected their decisions. The survey also asked about the process of searching for care, and how child care issues influence parents' careers and decision to stay in the military. Questions asking about how recent deployments affected child care arrangements were also included. The survey asked respondents to report on their family status. We report on the correspondence between reported family status and family status suggested by the data in the next section.

The sampling frame was developed according to data on active-duty military members and dependents from the Defense Manpower Data Center (DMDC). The sampling frame included all military members who reported having dependent children aged 12 years or younger as of September 2003. The DoD child-care-demand formula assigns a different probability that a family will "need" child care, depending on whether the military member is a single parent, the family is dual military, or the family has two adults, only one of whom is in the military.[1] Therefore, it was important for our study to get statistically significant estimates for each group separately.

Because we could not expect to achieve a large enough sample of single parents and dual military with a random sample, we used a clustered sample design, whereby we sampled single parents, dual-military, and "traditional" families (that is, military member married to a civilian spouse) separately. We pursued a stratified sample design by grouping military members by family status and child age. We had six separate sampling frames, and selected 500 families from each frame:

- single parents with children aged 0–5 years
- single parents with children aged 6–12 years
- dual military with children aged 0–5 years

---

[1] The DoD formula is detailed in Moini, Zellman, and Gates (2006).

- dual military with children aged 6–12 years
- traditional families with children aged 0–5 years
- traditional families with children aged 6–12 years.

We sampled without replacement, so that one family would not receive two surveys. Since it is possible for a military member to have children in both age ranges (0–5 years, 6–12 years), we first drew the sample for the group with children 0–5, then removed that family from both sampling frames.

Although we had been informed that DEERS data would enable us to identify dual-military spouses, in the course of this project we discovered that the DEERS file no longer includes a dual-military flag. Because it was important to survey dual-military families, and only a small number of such families would be reached through a random sample of military families, we asked DMDC to construct such a flag by looking for active-duty service members who report having spouses who are also active-duty service members (we looked for unique identifiers that indicate individuals as both sponsors (military members)[2] and dependent spouses).[3] Through this method, we identified approximately 10,000 dual-military families, which is about one-third of what we expected based on a comparison with other data sources. Because there is no requirement that service members report their dual-military spouses in DEERS, and because there is no financial incentive for them to do so, we are not surprised that the number of families in our dual-military file is smaller than other estimates of dual-military families.

Our survey sample included 3,000 military families. In February 2004, each family in the sample received an advance letter, signed by a senior official in their military service, announcing the survey and encouraging them to participate. This advance letter allowed us to identify some bad addresses before the initial survey was mailed out. We mailed surveys to families in mid-March, 2004. Reminder postcards were mailed at the end of March 2004. In April 2004, we obtained work email addresses for the military members and contacted them to verify home addresses and to encourage them to fill out the survey. A second survey packet was sent out in May 2005. Of the original sample, 355 members were deemed ineligible for the survey because of bad addresses or because we had mistakenly sampled two members of a dual-military couple (despite attempts to avoid doing that, as described above).

We selected a supplemental sample of 355 members and mailed surveys to those families at the end of May 2004. We closed the survey fielding in August 2004. No compensation was offered to survey respondents, consistent with DoD policy for DoD-sponsored surveys. In addition, telephone follow-up was precluded because DMDC data do not include

---

[2] The data set includes a record for each individual who is eligible for health insurance benefits under the military system. Individuals are eligible if they are a military member (they are the sponsor), or are the dependent spouse or child of a military member. Many people appear in the data set as both sponsors (military members) and dependent spouses of military members. We flag these individuals as dual military.

[3] Any unique identifier fitting that description appears in a "joint military couple" file. In some cases, we have pairs for which the active-duty husband claimed his wife and the active-duty wife claimed her husband. In other cases, only one spouse is claiming the other as a dependent spouse. We required only one spouse to claim the other in order to flag both spouses as "dual-military" sponsors. Any record that includes a sponsor flagged in this way is then included in the dual-military-family file, regardless of the marital status they report. There were a handful of individuals who reported a marital status of single and have a dependent child, but also appear in our dual-military couple file. We consider these individuals to be dual military, assuming this is an error in the reporting of marital status.

telephone numbers. We received a total of 1,137 responses to the survey, for a response rate of 34 percent.

Of the 1,137 survey responses, 109, or 10 percent, were parents who responded that the dependent child did not live with them and they had no input into the child care decisions for that child. Thus, our final analytic sample for the survey is 1,028.

Among those completing a survey, 12 percent are single parents, 44 percent are dual-military families, and 43 percent are military members married to civilians (1 percent were missing a response on this variable). One-third of the sampling frame was single parents, yet only 12 percent of completed surveys came from single parents. This disparity raises questions about the single-parent group. Analysis revealed that the very low fraction of single parents among survey respondents appears to be due not to low survey response rates among the people we had identified as single parents using DMDC data; rather, it is due to changes in family status among these individuals. Forty-five percent of those we had identified as single parents with a child between 0 and 5 years reported a different family status in their survey response. Similarly, 39 percent of those we had identified as a single parent with a child between 6 and 12 years reported a different family status on their survey form. The lack of correspondence works both ways, however: 8 percent of the survey respondents whom we had identified as married to civilians reported being single parents.

This rather high level of variation between family status reported in DMDC data and family status reported on the survey raises important issues for the use of DMDC data in the child-care-demand formula. It appears that family status is a moving target. Although the fact that there is a difference between marital status recorded in DEERS and that reported on the survey is not surprising—individuals may divorce and remarry—the magnitude of the difference for those identified in DEERS as single parents is striking (see Moini, Zellman, and Gates, 2006).

Weighting of Survey Responses

The results that we report in the next section are based on weighted survey data. Weighting is required to generate results that are representative of the DoD population as a whole. It allows us to account for our stratified sample design and for differences in response rates by service and military rank. The stratified sample design was used in order to ensure that the survey population captured a reasonable number of dual-military and single-parent families. The six strata, described earlier, are based on the age of the child (0–5 and 6–12 years) and on family status (single parent, dual military parents, or married to a civilian). We sampled 500 families from each of the six strata.[4]

Because the response rate is fairly low, we also developed weights to account for nonresponse. To develop the weights, we performed a logistic regression with survey response as the dependent variable and the following observable characteristics of sampled individuals as the independent variables: service, rank, Reserve indicator, gender, race (black, white, or other), years of service (under nine years of service or over nine years of service), and educa-

---

[4] Since the survey asks families about the child care arrangement for only one child, weights are constructed at the family level.

tion level (less than a B.A. or B.A. or higher). A complete description of this analysis is presented in Appendix B.

The analysis revealed that response rates were higher for Air Force personnel, officers, females, whites, and military members with a B.A. or higher.[5] The parameter estimates from the logistic regression were used to construct no-response weights. We combined the non-response weights with the sampling weights to produce an overall weight.

Analysis of Survey Results

In this report, we conduct multivariate analyses of survey results in order to better understand the relationships among individual family characteristics, characteristics of local installations, and child-care use patterns, as well as various measures of child care need.

Independent Variables Used in the Analysis

Judging from the discussion and hypotheses in the previous chapter, we expect that the following independent variables will influence the child care options that parents use. We include these variables as explanatory variables in the model. Table 3.1 summarizes the variables used in the analysis.

Family Status. The model includes a categorical variable describing the family status of the family. We allowed four options: the family is headed by a single military parent, it is a dual-military family in which both mother and father are in the military, the family consists of a military member married to a civilian spouse who works or attends school full- or part-time, and the family consists of a military member and a nonworking spouse. The omitted category in the analysis is single military parents.

Service. The model includes a categorical variable describing the military service of which the military member is a part. The three categorical variables included are Army, Navy, and Marine Corps.[6] Air Force is the omitted category in the regression analysis. When dual-military families include members of two different services, we coded the service of the mother (10 percent of dual-military families).

Total Family Income. The model includes a categorical variable describing the total family income. The four categories are less than $25,000, $25,000–$49,000, $50,000–$74,999, and $75,000 and above. The omitted category is $75,000 and above. Because few families with school-aged children fall into the lowest income category, we combined the two lower-income groups into one category for families earning less than $50,000 in the school-aged analysis.

Highest Rank of Military Parent. Because of the relatively small sample size, we did not include a detailed variable reflecting the highest rank of a military parent. Instead, we included an indicator variable reflecting whether at least one military parent is an officer or a warrant officer.

---

[5] The *p*-value associated with the chi-square statistic is 0.0000, indicating that the model as a whole is statistically significant. The pseudo *R*-square statistic for the model is .08.

[6] In some of the regression analyses, we were forced to combine Marine Corps and Navy into one Marine/Navy service category because of a small number of observations in the Marine Corps cell.

Table 3.1
Independent Variables Included in Regression Analyses

Variable name	Description
Single parent	Single military parent (omitted category)
Dual military	Dual-military parents
Working civilian spouse	Military parent with working civilian spouse
Nonworking civilian spouse	Military parent with nonworking civilian spouse
Air Force	Respondent is in the Air Force (omitted category)
Army	Respondent is in the Army
Navy	Respondent is in the Navy
Marines	Respondent is in the Marines
Navy/Marines	Respondent is in either the Marines or Navy
Family income <$25,000	Annual household income (2003) is less than $25,000 (in 2003 dollars)
Family income $25,000 to $49,999	Annual household income (2003) is between $25,000 and $49,999 (in 2003 dollars)
Family income $25,000 to $49,999	Annual household income (2003) is less than $50,000 (in 2003 dollars)
Family income $50,000 to $74,999	Annual household income (2003) is between $50,000 and $74,999 (in 2003 dollars)
Family income >$75,000	Annual household income (2003) is greater than $75,000 (in 2003 dollars) (omitted category)
Enlisted	Respondent is enlisted (omitted category)
Officer	Respondent is an officer
Child age is 0–5	Survey child is 0 to 5 years of age (omitted category)
Child age is 6–12	Survey child is 6 to 12 years of age
Child age is over 12	Survey child is at least 13 years of age
Lives on base	Respondent lives on base (omitted category)
Lives within 10 miles of base	Respondent lives off base, but within 10 miles of base
Lives 11 to 20 miles from base	Respondent lives 11 to 20 miles from base
Lives more than 20 miles from base	Respondent lives more than 20 miles from base
Reserves	Respondent is in the Reserves component
Family has another child aged 13–18	There is another child in the household aged 13 to 18
Work hours vary	Military parent has work hours that vary from week to week
Median income in local area	Median household income in zip code (per $1,000)
Children <age 6	Number of children under 6 years of age in the zip code
Children aged 6 to 12	Number of children 6 to 12 years of age in the zip code
Female unemployment rate	Female unemployment rate in the zip code
Local child-care supply	Total number of child care workers per number of <6-year-olds within 5 miles
Unmet need	Respondent experiences unmet child-care need
DoD CDC	Primary care provided by DoD child development center. (Omitted category in models focusing only on respondents with a child aged 0–5 years.)
DoD FCC	Primary care provided by DoD home or family child care
All DoD care	Primary care provided by DoD CDC, youth center, before- or after-school program, or DoD FCC
Formal civilian care	Primary care provided by civilian before- or after-school program, child care center, or family child care. (Omitted category in models focusing only on respondents with a child aged 6 through 12.)
Informal child care	Primary care provided by relative or nonrelative in or outside home, by older sibling, by child him-/herself, or other informal arrangement

Table 3.1
Continued

Variable name	Description
Parental care	Primary care provided by parent
Unmet preference	Family prefers another child care arrangement over the one they are using
Likely to leave military	Family is either very likely or somewhat likely to leave the armed services due to child care issues

Age of Sampled Child. For each analysis, we ran an overall model in which we combined survey responses from all families and included a dummy variable reflecting whether the child is aged 0–5 years, 6–12 years, or over 13 years. In these models, aged 0–5 years is the omitted category. We also ran regressions separately for responses related to children 0–5 and 6–12 years separately (we did not include children aged 13 plus in either regression). In most cases, the regression results differ by child age group, and we opted to report results separately. In summarizing the results, we also note whether the difference between pre–school- and school-aged children was statistically significant in the combined regression results.

How Far from Base the Family Lives. We include a categorical variable reflecting how far from base the family lives. It has four categories: live on base, live 1 to 10 miles from base, live between 11 and 20 miles, and live over 20 miles from base. Those living on base are the excluded category in the regression model. We expect those living closer to the base to be more likely to use DoD-sponsored child care.

Reserve Indicator. We include a categorical variable reflecting whether the military member is an activated Reservist. The variable takes on a value of 1 if the military member is in the Reserves and 0 otherwise.

Other Family Characteristics. We include an indicator variable that takes on a value of 1 if there is another child over age 12 in the family. We include this variable because families that have a child over age 13 in the household have an option of sibling care that is not available to other families.

We include an indicator variable reflecting whether the family reports that work hours of a military member vary from week to week.

Characteristics of the Local Community. To characterize the local community, we link 2000 census data to the survey data by zip code. We include in the models data on the median household income in the zip code, the female unemployment rate, and the number of child care workers per child between the ages of 0 and 6 years. Median income is a rough measure of the wealth of the local community. The income of military families does not vary much by location. If the price of non-DoD child-care options is higher in areas in which the median family income is higher, then we would expect those child care options to be relatively more costly for military families in areas where the median income is higher. The female unemployment rate is included to reflect the local labor-market conditions that civilian spouses face. We might expect parental care to be more common in areas in which the female unemployment rate is higher. Finally, following Gordon and Chase-Lansdale (2001), we create a rough measure of the child care supply in the local community by dividing the number of child care workers within a 5-mile radius of the zip code of the installation by the number of children aged 0–6 years. Our ability to match survey responses to census data was limited by the fact that the census files do not provide information on the aforementioned criteria for low-population areas.[7] As a result, we lose some observations in the analysis when we include the census variables. However, by running the models with and without these variables, we do not notice a change in the statistical significance of the parameter estimates due to the inclusion or exclusion of these variables. This lack of change suggests that the survey observations that we lose due to a lack of zip-code information do not differ in systematic ways from the observations that remain. This finding gives us more confidence in reporting the results that include these independent variables, in spite of the fact that we lose observations.

Type of Care Used by the Family. In the regression analysis that examines unmet preference and the likelihood that the family reports a propensity to leave the military due to child care issues, we include among the explanatory variables a categorical variable reflecting the type of care that the family uses. The categories differ for the 0–5 age group and the 6–12 age group. Our survey allowed parents to choose from among 17 possible child-care options. Because of the small number of survey responses, it is necessary to group the child care options into a smaller number of categories in order to support an econometric analysis of the data. For pre–school-aged children, we collapse these choices into four possible outcome categories: DoD CDC (includes the handful of responses for DoD school-aged care and youth center), DoD FCC, formal civilian child-care options (civilian after-school program, civilian child-care center, and civilian FCC) and informal civilian child-care options (includes relative care, nonrelative care, sibling care, and self-care). The number of families using CDC and DoD FCC care for school-aged children is small; therefore, we include only three possible outcome categories, grouping all DoD-sponsored child care options (including FCC) into one category.

Analysis of Unmet Need

The purpose of these analyses is to better understand the factors that relate to the probability that a family experiences *unmet need,* defined as families who use any informal care arrangement (such as relative or nonrelative in or outside of the home) or parental, sibling, or self-care *and* report that they would prefer another option. To analyze unmet need, we used a probit model framework to estimate the relationship between family and installation characteristics and the probability that a family experiences unmet need. We include the explanatory variables discussed in the preceding section.

---

[7] Out of the 1,028 survey response observations, 585 (57 percent) merged perfectly with census data, leaving 443 (43 percent) that did not have these new census variables matched to them. Some of the zip codes in the census file ended in XX, all of which are low-population areas. In an attempt to match the 443 that did not match in the first round, we recoded those census zips with XX on the end to have 00 on the end (for example, 905XX becomes 90500). The unmatched zip codes also had the last two digits recoded to 00 (90512 becomes 90500). With the recodes, we tried to merge the zips together. This time around, 151 observations matched to the new census data, leaving 292 that do not match to the census data. The newly matched 151 observations now have all the census variables attached to them, except for total number of child care workers, because it could not be calculated for the zip codes ending in 00. These zip codes do not have a centroid attached to them, and geographic information systems (GIS) software needs a centroid in order to be able to calculate a distance measure (5 miles, 10 miles, etc.). Therefore, 292 (30 percent) observations do not have any of the new census variables and 151 (15 percent) have all but total child-care workers. We then used the hotdeck imputation method to reassign zip codes to those that did not match. This method assigns a new zip code at random. Once that was done, we remerged the new census variables using the new zip codes. Imputing the zip codes allows us to keep the census variables together by zip code. If we were to impute the census variables separately, then it is possible to assign an unmatched zip code a value for median income from one zip code and a value for number of children under 6 years from another. We avoid this by imputing the whole zip code.

Analysis of Unmet Preference

Many families are using a formal child-care arrangement that is not their first choice. These families cannot be described as having unmet need, because they do have access to an arrangement that allows one or both parents to work. However, these families report that they would prefer to be using a different option. We use a probit model framework to estimate the relationship between family and installation characteristics and the probability that a family reports unmet child-care preference. We include the same explanatory variables discussed above in the description of the model of unmet need. In addition, we include a categorical variable reflecting the primary child-care arrangement used by the family.

Analysis of Families Likely to Leave the Military Due to Child Care Issues

As an employer, DoD may be particularly concerned about families who report that they are likely to leave the military because of challenges with child care. We use a probit model framework to estimate the relationship between family and installation characteristics and the probability that a family reports that they are likely or very likely to leave the military due to child care issues.

We include the same explanatory variables discussed above in the description of the model of unmet need. In addition, we include a categorical variable reflecting the primary child-care arrangement used by the family.

Child Care Choice

To analyze child care choice, we use a two-stage approach. First, we use a probit model to analyze the probability that a family uses parental care or not. Then, we use a multinomial logit model to examine the child care choice among families that use a nonparental care option as their primary method of child care.[8] The multinomial logit model is a common approach for examining the choice among several different options (Allison, 1982, 1984). In this analysis the dependent variable is the same as the independent variable used to reflect child care choice in other analyses, such as the analysis of unmet preference. For pre–school-aged children, we collapse these choices into four possible outcome categories: DoD CDC, DoD FCC, formal civilian child-care options, and informal civilian child-care options. For school-aged children, we include only three possible outcome categories, grouping all DoD-sponsored child-care options (including FCC) into one category.

Multinomial logit models simultaneously examine the probability that the family chooses each option and describe the odds of being in one category instead of another. The values of the regression coefficients indicate the effect of the predictor (on one outcome relative to the baseline category), after controlling for all other predictors; these are partial regression coefficients. The associated p-value indicates whether the regression coefficient value is statistically significantly different from zero. In summarizing the results of the regression analysis, we discuss parameter estimates as significant if the p-value is less than .05.

---

[8] We also explored an alternative one-stage modeling structure reflecting a simultaneous choice among parental and nonparental options. Specifically, we estimated a five-category multinomial logit model. The Hausman-McFadden test indicated that, under this model structure, the data violate the independence of irrelevant alternatives (IIA) assumption. The second stage of the two-stage model, the results of which are reported here, satisfies the IIA assumptions. We also considered using a nested logit modeling approach; however, we had no conceptual basis on which to group the various child-care choices into nests.

Unfortunately, these parameter estimates do not allow for an intuitive interpretation of the results. Although we can say with confidence that a parameter estimate is statistically significantly different from zero, the magnitude of the coefficient does not provide much insight into how important, or "big," the effect is. To get a sense of how important the results are, we examine the predicted response probability, which gives the probability of occurrence for an event. To calculate the predicted probability, values of the covariates must be selected. The model may be used to predict values for the "average" person or for specific policy-relevant characteristics.

One option for generating these predicted probabilities is to fix the values of continuous and categorical covariates at their sample means (see Gates et al., 2004). These means are what an "average" person in the existing sample may look like, because these values represent the marginal distributions of covariates in the present sample. Substituting these covariate values produces a predicted probability for an "average" family.

We were also interested in calculating probabilities in order to describe the effect of statistically significant explanatory variables in all models. For example, consider the dummy variables used to identify family type. To calculate the probability of a particular outcome for a dual-military family, we plug in values of 1 for the dual-military dummy and 0 for the single-parent and married-to-civilian dummies. We then calculate the predicted probability while holding all other values for the independent variables fixed at their sample means. This process can be compared with parallel calculations for single-parent families and families with a civilian spouse. Using a similar approach, it is also possible to explore the effects of other dummy variables. In the Results chapter, Chapter 4, we present such probability estimations in tabular form after the tables containing coefficient estimates.

An important assumption of the multinomial logit model is the independence of irrelevant alternatives (IIA). This assumption states that the relative probability of any two outcomes is not altered by the inclusion of other possible outcomes. In our case, such an assumption implies that the relative probability of using formal civilian child care over DoD FCC is not influenced by whether or not DoD CDC care is an option. We might be concerned, for example, that unobserved characteristics of individuals that make them more likely to use DoD CDC care might also make them more or less likely to use formal civilian-care options if DoD CDC care is not available.

A test for the IIA assumption, based on Hausman and McFadden (1984), is available in STATA.[9] The premise of the test is that if IIA is a valid assumption, then dropping one category from the model should not change the estimated coefficients. Applied to the model of child care choice, the test supports the validity of the IIA assumption in our application, except with respect to the use of the "informal care" group, suggesting that the model is appropriate for the consideration of the probability of using forms of care other than informal care.

---

[9] STATA is a standard statistical software package. It is available through www.stata.com.

CHAPTER FOUR

Results

In this chapter, we provide an overview of the survey responses, focusing on issues of relevance to the DoD's child-care-demand formula and our analysis of child care need. We also discuss the results of our analyses of four major outcomes of interest: unmet need, unmet preference, propensity to leave the military because of child care issues, and child care choice.

Overview of Survey Responses

As mentioned in Chapter Two, 13 percent of families who returned surveys reported that the target child does not live with them and that they are not involved in their child care decisions. An additional 3 percent of those who completed the survey reported that the child does not live with them. Thus, 16 percent of our survey respondents indicated that a randomly selected minor dependent does not live with them, but a quarter of those respondents are involved in child care decisions and completed our survey.

As expected, there were strong differences across family type in the fraction of parents who reported that their target child does not live with them. Thirty-one percent of single parents, less than 1 percent of dual-military parents, and 15 percent of married-to-civilian families reported that the target dependent child in question did not live with them.

Table 4.1 reflects the survey respondents' reports of typical child-care arrangements for the sample child, by child age (0–5 and 6–12 years). One observation that follows immediately from Table 4.1 is that, as expected, military families are far less likely than U.S. families as a whole to use relative or sibling care. As we noted in Chapter 2, approximately one-third of civilian families with a working mother use some form of relative care.

Characteristics of Survey Respondents

A majority (61 percent) of survey respondents reported that work hours vary from week to week.

Only 28 percent of respondents live on base. Most (73 percent) live within 20 miles of the installation. The main reasons for living off base are the quality of housing/school/neighborhood and the desire to buy a home.

Of families who have been deployed, 18 percent report some change in child care arrangements was needed during the last deployment. However, only 25 percent of those

Table 4.1
Primary Child-Care Arrangement, by Child Age (Percentage)

Arrangement	Aged 0–5 years	Aged 6–12 years	All[a]
DoD CDC	16.20	1.35	7.03
DoD FCC	10.06	0.55	4.24
DoD school-aged care	0.06	1.67	0.79
DoD youth center	1.01	4.08	2.17
DoD after-school program	0	2.88	1.00
Civilian after-school program	0.63	9.19	3.76
Civilian child-care center	12.94	3.45	6.87
Civilian family child care	3.66	0.65	2.16
Relative	4.28	5.66	6.44
Parent	33.76	45.56	34.58
Sibling	0	0.36	3.02
Nonrelative	5.64	3.19	5.36
Other or missing	10.08	7.36	19.94
N	463	415	1,028

[a]All responses include those from families who did not report the age of the child or for which the age of the child was over 12.

families who experienced a change reported that it was difficult or very difficult to get child care after the deployment ended.

Among those who do not rely on anyone beyond a parent to care for the child, more than half (68 percent) have a spouse who does not work outside the home or is self-employed. Twelve percent report that they take advantage of flexible work hours or that parents work different shifts.

Among civilian spouses of military members, over half (56 percent) are employed or attending school full- or part-time. Over half of survey respondents agree or strongly agree that work opportunities for civilian spouses are limited (57 percent) and that good opportunities require a long commute (58 percent). Very few (less than 5 percent) "strongly disagree" with these statements.

Child Care and Military Readiness

Child care issues do appear to influence the readiness of military members, and the effect of such issues appears to be greater for female military members than for males. Among families with a military father, 23 percent of survey respondents reported that the military father was late to work due to child care issues in the last month. This lateness tended to happen one or two times in the past month; however, for some, it happened up to 20 times. For families with a military mother, 51 percent reported that the military mother was late to work due to child care issues. Similarly, among families with a military father, 7 percent of survey respondents reported that the military father missed work due to child care issues in the past month. For families with a military mother, the figure was 37 percent. Clearly, military women are carrying a bigger load of the child care burden; they cover for child care inadequacies more than do male military members.

What Survey Responses Reflect in Terms of Child Care Need

Nearly 9 percent of parents have *unmet need* according to the definition we discussed earlier in this report. This figure includes families who use any informal care arrangement (such as relative or nonrelative in or outside of the home) or parental, sibling, or self-care *and* report that they would prefer another option. This is a fairly broad definition of *unmet need,* but the more-restrictive definitions we explored (e.g., including only parents who use parental, sibling, or self-care) captured very few families. Note that the definition of *unmet need* does not include families who are currently using some sort of formal child-care arrangement, even if they report that it is not their preferred option. So, for example, families using DoD FCC who would prefer to have their child in a CDC are not characterized as having unmet need. Similarly, unmet need does not include families who are using an informal arrangement or parental care, unless they also report that they would prefer some other option. Parents of pre–school-aged children are neither more nor less likely than parents of school-aged children to experience unmet need.

In addition to the concept of unmet need, we also explore *unmet preference* in this report. Families experiencing unmet preference are those who report that their current child-care arrangement is not their first choice, regardless of what type of care it is. Twenty-six percent of survey respondents replied that they would prefer another child care arrangement. Parents of pre–school-aged children appear to be more likely to report unmet preference (29.90 percent) than do parents of school-aged children (18.71 percent).

For those with pre–school-aged children, the most favored alternatives are DoD CDC (51 percent), DoD FCC (5 percent), and relative care (14 percent). After-school programs (both DoD and civilian) are most preferred by those with school-aged children (37 percent), followed by relative care (17 percent) and nonrelative care (11 percent). If we group DoD school-aged, youth program, and after-school programs with DoD CDC, the total unmet preference for structured DoD programs would be 30 percent. Among those who express unmet preference for some DoD-sponsored child care, the vast majority (71 percent) is not currently using DoD-sponsored child care.

Although many parents are expressing a preference for DoD-sponsored care, many families who currently use DoD-sponsored care are stating a preference for some other form of care. Differences among DoD FCC users, DoD CDC users, and those using formal civilian-care options are not statistically significant, indicating that these groups seem about as likely to say that they would prefer another option (48 percent, 29 percent, and 31 percent, respectively).

Another way of thinking about whether existing child-care options are meeting the needs of military families is to consider whether families are forced to cobble together multiple care arrangements to ensure an adequate amount of continuous care for their children. Of the families that responded, 19 percent reported using more than one child care arrangement in the past week. Only 3 percent of families reported using more than one additional arrangement. Among families who used one or more additional arrangements, a vast majority (66 percent of those reporting an additional arrangement) used additional arrangements for 10 or fewer hours per week. These "other arrangements" tend to be informal ones: relatives or nonrelatives in-home or outside the home.

A final measure of whether DoD is meeting the child care needs of military families is reflected in whether families report that child care concerns might drive them to *leave the military*. Twenty-one percent of families reported that it is likely or very likely that they will leave the military due to child care issues. Forty-two percent reported that it is very unlikely. Families with pre–school-aged children appear much more likely to report that they will leave the service due to child care issues (35.72 percent) compared with parents of school-aged children (15.13 percent).

In the analyses that follow, we focus on the factors that relate to three conceptions of child care need: unmet need, unmet preference, and propensity to report plans to leave the military. We also analyze the choice among different care options.

Unmet Need

Nearly 9 percent of parents responding to the survey reported having unmet need. A combined regression reveals that families are more likely to report unmet need for children between the ages of 0 and 5 years than for older children.[1] Table 4.2 reports the results of the probit regression coefficients from analysis of unmet need among families with children aged 0 through 5 years. As mentioned in Chapter Three, the parameter estimates for these models do not have a straightforward interpretation. However, the table does help the reader identify the independent variables that have a statistically significant relationship with the dependent variable (p-value is less than .05) and to determine the direction of that relationship.

We use the parameter estimates in Table 4.2 to conduct probability calculations as described in Chapter 3. These probabilities are summarized in Table 4.2a. We find that dual-military families are 7 percentage points less likely than single parents to report unmet need, whereas parents of military members with civilian working spouses are 4 percentage points more likely than single parents to report unmet need. This difference accords with our hypothesis that the preference given to dual-military and single-parent families in the DoD child-care system would result in less unmet need among these families.

The analysis also suggests that the income level of the military family relates to reports of unmet need. Compared with families that had earnings greater than $75,000 in 2003, those earning less than $50,000 per year were more likely to report unmet need. Families earning less than $25,000 per year were 4 percentage points more likely, and families earning between $25,000 and $50,000 per year were 18 percentage points more likely, to report unmet need.

Among families of children between the ages of 6 and 12 years, we find no statistically significant relationship between family or installation characteristics and report of unmet need, as reflected in Table 4.2. This finding is likely due to two phenomena: So few families with children in this age range report any unmet need, and, within various covariate categories, few observations expressed unmet need.[2]

Unmet Preference

Although relatively few families report unmet child-care need (9 percent), they are more than twice as likely (22 percent) to report unmet preference. As with unmet need, families are more likely to express unmet preference for care for younger children, aged 0 through 5

---

[1] We do not report the results of the combined regressions here, but results are available from the authors upon request.

[2] Specifically, only 18 families with children in this age range expressed unmet need. If we break this number down by family type, only three single-parent families, seven dual-military families, six civilian families with a working spouse, and two families with a civilian nonworking spouse expressed unmet need. Other categorical variables suffer from similar problems.

Table 4.2
Unmet Child-Care Need for Pre–School-Aged and School-Aged Children

Unmet need variable name	Pre–school-aged children		School-aged children	
	Coefficient	Standard error	Coefficient	Standard error
Dual military	−2.1959***	0.7230	0.5084	0.8253
Working civilian spouse	0.3440	0.5463	0.6427	0.6077
Nonworking civilian spouse	0.7941	0.5191	−0.3783	0.6145
Work hours vary	0.3235	0.3492	0.3615	0.3748
Family income <$25,000	2.2119**	0.9361		
Family income <$50,000			0.7978	0.6264
Family income $25,000 to $49,999	3.4262***	0.8418		
Family income $50,000 to $74,999	1.8605**	0.7820	−0.8678	0.7285
Lives within 10 miles of base	0.5145	0.4289	0.2830	0.4677
Lives 11 to 20 miles from base	−0.0602	0.5817	−0.0651	0.5101
Lives >20 miles from base	−0.1951	0.5103	0.9830	0.6401
Officer	1.5792*	0.8419	0.8442	0.6194
Army	−0.4601	0.5208	−0.3141	0.4958
Navy/Marines	−1.1362	0.9279	−0.1760	0.5203
Reserves	−1.1362	0.9279	0.1042	0.6986
Median income in local area	−0.0000	0.0322	0.0200	0.0201
Female unemployment rate	0.0406	0.0463	−0.0737	0.0669
Local child–care supply	−0.0270	0.0374	−0.0020	0.0135
Constant	−4.7132***	1.4065	−2.7734***	0.8627
	$N = 296$		$N = 263$	
	$F(17,590) = 3.15$		$F(16,591) = 1.17$	
	Prob $> F = 0.0000$		Prob $> F = 0.2893$	

Significance levels: *** 0.01 level, ** 0.05 level, * 0.10 level.

Table 4.2a
Predicted Probability of Expressing Unmet Child-Care Need

Variable name	Pre–school-aged children	School-aged children
Family type		
Dual military	0.01***	0.13
Working civilian spouse	0.12	0.15
Nonworking civilian spouse	0.19	0.03
Single military parent^	0.08	0.06
Family income		
<$25,000	0.05**	
<$50,000		0.09
$25,000 to $49,999	0.19***	
$50,000 to $74,999	0.03**	0.24
$75,000+^	0.01	0.02

^ indicates that this is the omitted category in the regression model.
Asterisks reflect that the predicted probability for this category is significantly different from that of the omitted category: *** 0.01 level, ** 0.05 level, * 0.10 level.

years. Table 4.3 presents the regression results for the analysis of unmet preference among families with pre–school-aged children.

Our probability calculations, summarized in Table 4.3a, suggest that among parents of pre–school-aged children, those whose work hours vary are 22 percentage points more likely to report unmet preference. This suggests that available child-care arrangements may not match well with irregular military schedules. Relative to Air Force families, Army and Marine Corps families are substantially less likely (21 percentage points and 39 percentage points, respectively) to report unmet child-care preference.

Table 4.3a also presents the results of a probit regression analysis of unmet preference for families with school-aged children. Our probability calculations based on these results reveal that, among parents of school-aged children, those using DoD-sponsored arrangements were 39 percentage points less likely than those using civilian-run formal care to express unmet preference. Similarly, those using parental care were 41 percentage points less likely than those using formal civilian options to express unmet preference. This table suggests that families using civilian-run formal care for their school-aged children are most likely to express unmet preference. This result may be due to a lack of DoD-sponsored child care for school-aged children or to logistical barriers that render DoD-sponsored options inconvenient for many families.

Indeed, our focus group discussions revealed that some parents cannot use DoD-sponsored school-aged care because of a lack of transportation between the school and the DoD program. Dual-military families with school-aged children are 61 percentage points

Table 4.3
Unmet Child-Care Preference for Pre–School-Aged and School-Aged Children

Unmet preference variable name	Pre–school-aged children		School-aged children	
	Coefficient	Standard error	Coefficient	Standard error
Dual military	0.1674	0.5207	2.4243***	0.6863
Working civilian spouse	−0.0558	0.4253	0.8553*	0.4941
Nonworking civilian spouse	0.3401	0.4270	−0.2474	0.6346
Work hours vary	0.6860**	0.3095	0.7585**	0.3292
Family income <$25,000	0.1882	0.8340		
Family income <$50,000			0.3790	0.6029
Family income $25,000 to $49,999	0.5860	0.7749		
Family income $50,000 to $74,999	0.0372	0.7164	−0.6269	0.5193
Lives within 10 miles of base	−0.1235	0.4175	−0.1748	0.4828
Lives 11 to 20 miles from base	−0.6384**	0.4885	−0.3481	0.4382
Lives >20 miles from base	0.0554	0.4597	0.1823	0.5677
Officer	0.6299	0.7265	0.1455	0.5734
Army	−0.6666*	0.3995	−0.2530	0.4254
Navy	−0.5532	0.4019		
Marines	−1.5345**	0.6165		
Navy/Marines			−0.2865	0.4447
All DoD care			−1.6305***	0.5519
DoD FCC	0.6066	0.5756		
Parental care	−0.0524	0.4638	−1.7557***	0.5209
Formal civilian care	0.5977	0.4777		
Informal child care	0.1518	0.5507	−1.3790***	0.4598
Reserves	−0.8441	0.7624	0.0807	0.7444
Median income in local area	−0.0232	0.0214	0.0268	0.0187
Female unemployment rate	−0.0230	0.0393	0.0352	0.0447
Local child-care supply	−0.0076	0.0117	−0.0190	0.0413
	$N = 296$		$N = 263$	
	$F (22,585) = 1.16$		$F (19,588) = 5.32$	
	Prob > F = 0.0819		Prob > F = 0.0000	

Significance levels: *** 0.01 level, ** 0.05 level, * 0.10 level.

Table 4.3a
Predicted Probability of Expressing Unmet Child-Care Preference

Variable name	Pre–school-aged children	School-aged children
Family type		
Dual military	0.42	0.73***
Working civilian spouse	0.35	0.28*
Nonworking civilian spouse	0.48	0.09
Single military parent^	0.37	0.12
Work hours vary week to week		
Yes	0.49**	0.47**
No^	0.27	0.32
Distance between home and base		
Lives on base^	0.47	0.43
10 miles or less	0.43	0.40
11–20 miles	0.28**	0.36
More than 20 miles	0.49	0.47
Service		
Air Force^	0.49	0.43
Army	0.28*	0.38
Navy	0.32	
Marine Corps	0.10**	
Navy/Marine Corps		0.37
Type of child care		
All DoD		0.30***
DoD FCC	0.54	
Parental care	0.32	0.28***
Formal civilian care^	0.53	0.69
Informal child care	0.39	0.36***
DoD CDC^	0.34	

^ indicates that this is the omitted category in the regression model. For type of child care, DoD CDC is the omitted category for pre–school-aged children only. Formal civilian care is the omitted category for school-aged children.

Asterisks reflect that the predicted probability for this category is significantly different from that of the omitted category: *** 0.01 level, ** 0.05 level, * 0.10 level.

more likely than single parents to report unmet preference. Finally, families who have variable work hours were more likely than families with regular work hours to report unmet preference.[3]

Likelihood of Leaving the Military

Families with pre–school-aged children were much more likely than families with school-aged children to report a propensity to leave the military. This difference may be partially due to the fact that the parents of older children tend to be older themselves and to have a longer tenure in and stronger commitment to the military career.

Our analyses suggest that family status and service-related differences have a strong relationship with plans to leave the service for families with pre–school-aged children. Table 4.4 presents the results of the probit analysis for these families. Table 4.4a summarizes the relationship between statistically significant independent variables and the probability that a military member expresses a propensity to leave the military due to child care issues.

Among families with pre–school-aged children, military members with civilian non-working spouses are 19 percentage points less likely to be considering leaving the military due to child care issues than are single military parents. This makes sense, given that a parent at home caring for children is the most flexible arrangement possible. Further, in most cases, it is reasonable to assume that a nonworking parent is a choice the family makes to handle child care. On the other hand, dual-military families were nearly 30 percentage points more likely than single parents to report that child care issues were leading them to consider leaving the military. There was no statistically significant difference between single parents and military members with civilian working spouses, which suggests that, despite policies that favor single parents and dual military in CDC enrollment, dual-military parents still find it difficult to balance military work for both parents and family demands. Our survey question did not specifically ask whether one or both parents was likely to leave the military due to child care issues, simply how likely it was that the "family" would leave the military due to child care issues. For dual-military couples, the term *family* may have been interpreted to mean that one of the two parents is likely to leave the military. Indeed, our focus group participants included many "military married to civilian" families in which the civilian spouse had been a member of the military at one time.

---

[3] At the suggestion of a reviewer, we reran the models of unmet preference, using a narrower definition of the term that excludes families that have unmet need. The models change a bit structurally, because all people who are using parental care or informal care drop out of the models, by definition. For the independent variables that remain, we can compare the results of the models with and without people who expressed unmet need.

For pre–school-aged children, the results are more or less the same. The only change is that Army families are less likely to express this type of unmet preference, and Marine Corps families are not statistically significantly different from Air Force families. For school-aged children, the results differ in several ways from the results that use the broader definition of unmet *preference*. First, dual-military families no longer differ from other families in terms of the probability that they express unmet preference. Secondly, income variables are significant, suggesting that lower-income families are substantially less likely to express unmet preference conditional on no unmet need. Third, we find that families who live off base, but within 10 miles of base, are significantly less likely than those on base to express unmet preference conditional on no unmet need. The parameter estimate on the Reserve indicator is also positive, suggesting that Reservists are more likely to express unmet preference conditional on no unmet need.

Table 4.4
Propensity to Leave the Military for Pre–School- and School-Aged Children

Leaving variable name	Pre–school-aged children		School-aged children	
	Coefficient	Standard error	Coefficient	Standard error
Dual military	1.068*	0.6030	–0.0959	0.6270
Working civilian spouse	–0.5482	0.4378	–0.9700**	0.4722
Nonworking civilian spouse	–0.7347	0.4620	–0.8949	0.5686
Work hours vary	–0.5651*	0.3175	–0.0114	0.3689
Family income <$25,000	0.1651	0.7122		
Family income $25,000 to $49,999	0.1827	0.6328		
Family income <$50,000			–0.9356	0.6164
Family income $50,000 to $74,999	–0.1348	0.6460	–4.4341***	0.7263
Lives within 10 miles of base	0.2680	0.4773	0.1906	0.4345
Lives 11 to 20 miles from base	0.4518	0.5242	0.5855	0.5307
Lives >20 miles from base	0.5694	0.4826	1.2895**	0.6190
Officer	–1.0985*	0.6357	–1.4657**	0.6860
Army	0.6001	0.4499	0.4286	0.4296
Navy	0.1015	0.4539		
Marines	–0.5905	0.5951		
Navy/Marines			–0.2737	0.5233
DoD FCC	–1.6780***	0.5721		
All DoD care			–0.5132	0.6749
Parental care	–1.2150***	0.4454	–1.2799**	0.5646
Formal civilian care	–0.6634	0.4786		
Informal child care	–0.8234	0.4888	–1.8250***	0.5702
Reserves	–0.1436	0.6300	1.6727**	0.7503
Median income in local area	0.0137	0.0209	–0.0506	0.0322
Female unemployment rate	–0.1067**	0.0495	–0.0574	0.0425
Local child-care supply	0.0084	0.0080	0.0167***	0.0054
Constant	1.0077	1.0437	2.7638**	1.2272
	N = 294		N = 261	
	F (22,579) = 3.03		F (19,582) = 4.05	
	Prob > F = 0.0000		Prob > F = 0.0000	

Significance levels: *** 0.01 level, ** 0.05 level, * 0.10 level.

Table 4.4a
Predicted Probability of Expressing a Propensity to Leave the Military Due to Child Care Issues

Variable name	Pre–school-aged children	School-aged children
Family type		
Dual military	0.71*	0.30
Working civilian spouse	0.26	0.16**
Nonworking civilian spouse	0.22	0.17
Single military parent^	0.41	0.32
Work hours vary week to week		
Yes	0.48*	0.25
No^	0.62	0.25
Family income		
<$25,000	0.55	
<$50,000		0.27
$25,000 to $49,999	0.56	
$50,000 to $74,999	0.48	0.02***
$75,000+^	0.51	0.48
Distance between home and base		
Lives on base^	0.45	0.18
10 miles or less	0.51	0.21
11–20 miles	0.56	0.28
More than 20 miles	0.59	0.41**
Rank		
Officer	0.39*	0.16**
Enlisted^	0.65	0.37
Reservist		
Yes	0.50	0.53**
No^	0.53	0.21**
Type of child care		
All DoD		0.32
DoD FCC	0.24***	
Parental care	0.36***	0.18**
Formal civilian care^	0.52*	0.43
Informal child care	0.47**	0.11***
DoD CDC^	0.71	

Table 4.4a
Continued

Variable name	Pre–school-aged children	School-aged children
Local female unemployment rate		
25th percentile	0.63**	0.30
75th percentile	0.48**	0.24
Local child-care supply		
25th percentile	0.52	0.24***
75th percentile	0.53	0.25***

^ indicates that this is the omitted category in the regression model. For type of child care, DoD CDC is the omitted category for pre–school-aged children only. Formal civilian care is the omitted category for school-aged children.
Asterisks reflect that the predicted probability for this category is significantly different from that of the omitted category or that the relationship between the dependent variable and the independent variable is statistically different from zero: *** 0.01 level, ** 0.05 level, * 0.10 level.

The type of child care arrangement currently used also relates to reports of the likelihood of leaving the service. Compared with families using the DoD CDC, families using all other care arrangements, including DoD FCC, are substantially *less* likely to report that they are considering leaving the military due to child care issues. Note that these analyses control for family type, so these differences should not be driven by the fact that dual-military families are more likely to use the CDC and also are more likely to state a propensity to leave the military. Families using DoD FCC are 47 percentage points less likely, families using parental care are 35 percentage points less likely, those using informal care arrangements are 24 percentage points less likely than families using the CDC to report a propensity to leave the military. The results also suggest that families of military officers are less likely to report that they have considered leaving the military due to child care issues than are families of enlisted personnel.

Table 4.4a presents similar results for families with school-aged children. Among families of school-aged children, there was no statistically significant difference in the probability that a family is considering leaving the military by family type. Relative to families using formal civilian child-care options, those using civilian informal care are less likely to report a propensity to leave the military. Income characteristics and officer status also appear to influence this probability. Relative to families with incomes over $100,000 per year, families with lower incomes are less likely to report a propensity to leave the military. Officers with school-aged children are also less likely than enlisted families to report a likelihood of leaving the military. Reservists with school-aged children are more likely to report having considered leaving the service.

We reran the models described in Table 4.4, including "unmet preference" as an explanatory variable. In these models, the parameter estimate on unmet preference is positive and highly statistically significant, suggesting that families that express unmet preference are also much more likely to say that child care issues are leading them to consider leaving the military. Probability calculations using the results from this model suggest that, among families with pre–school-aged children, families that express unmet preference are 21 percentage points more likely to say that they plan to leave the military due to child care issues. Families of school-aged children who express unmet preference are 23 percentage points more likely to say that they plan to leave the military.

Child Care Choice

In modeling child care choice, we first consider the question of whether a family uses parental care or not, and then for those families who do not use parental care, we explore the question of which child care option they choose. Not surprisingly, the factors that influence the decision to use parental care differ from the factors influencing the type of care used, and the factors differ by child age.

Decision to Use Parental Care. Table 4.5 presents the results of the probit regression analysis of the probability that a family uses parental care, for families with children aged 0 through 5 years. Table 4.5a presents the associated probability calculations for statistically significant variables. Compared with single military parents, dual-military families are 9 percentage points less likely to use parental care, and civilian families with nonworking or working spouses are more likely to use parental care (53 percentage points and 33 percentage points, respectively). Families who live off base but within 10 miles of the installation are 14 percentage points more likely than those on base to use parental care. Families who live in a community with a greater supply of child care workers are less likely to use parental care for their pre–school-aged children, which is consistent with our hypothesis that, in areas in which the supply of non-DoD child-care options is greater, civilian spouses are more likely to work outside the home and use that care.

Table 4.5a presents similar results for families with school-aged children. Compared with single military parents, dual-military families are 34 percentage points less likely to use parental care, and civilian families with nonworking spouses are 34 percentage points more likely to use parental care. Families with incomes less than $50,000 per year and families with incomes of more than $100,000 per year are more likely to use parental care than are families whose income is between $75,000 and $100,000. Families whose highest-ranking military member is an officer are more likely that families of enlisted personnel to use parental care for their school-aged children. Finally, families living in areas with higher median incomes are more likely to use parental care for their school-aged children. Families living in a community at the 75th percentile of income are 9 percentage points more likely to use parental care than those living in a community at the 25th percentile of income, all else being equal.

Choice Among Nonparental Care Options. Table 4.6 presents the results of the multinomial logit analysis of child care choice. The table reports coefficient estimates. A negative value for the coefficient means that higher values of the independent variable (or, in the case of categorical variables, the fact that the family falls into that category rather than the omitted category) are associated with a lower relative probability of using that type of child care than CDC care (or, for school-aged children, any DoD care). A positive

Table 4.5
Use of Parental Care for Pre–School- and School-Aged Children

Parent	Pre–school-aged children		School-aged children	
	Coefficient	Standard error	Coefficient	Standard error
Family has another child aged 13–18			0.0960	0.5011
Dual military	−1.0032	0.7565	−1.9041***	0.5264
Working civilian spouse	1.3454**	0.5916	−0.2075	0.4535
Nonworking civilian spouse	2.0418***	0.5741	1.0939***	0.4535
Work hours vary	−0.2222	0.3215	−0.1066	0.3001
Family income <$25,000	−0.7988	0.8991		
Family income $25,000 to $49,999	0.3338	0.7327		
Family income <$50,000			1.1514**	0.4970
Family income $50,000 to $74,999	−1.0370	0.7246	−0.0763	0.4080
Lives within 10 miles of base	0.9910**	0.4125	0.3434	0.4068
Lives 11 to 20 miles from base	0.3143	0.5608	−0.1822	0.3972
Lives >20 miles from base	0.3143	0.5608	0.2407	0.4207
Officer	0.1356	0.4742	0.8822*	0.4974
Army	−0.1841	0.4574	0.3777	0.3643
Navy	0.3089	0.4087	0.0243	0.3559
Marines	0.5299	0.8513	0.8659	0.6585
Reserves	0.2592	0.6442	0.2924	0.5104
Median income in local area	−0.0219	0.0317	0.0585**	0.0255
Female unemployment rate	−0.0200	0.0425	−0.0236	0.0293
Local child-care supply	−0.1374**	0.0687	0.0161*	0.0083
Constant	−1.1669	1.3679	−2.6988***	0.9935
	N = 323		N = 285	
	$F(18,643) = 3.12$		$F(18,643) = 6.69$	
	Prob > F = 0.0000		Prob > F = 0.0000	

Significance levels: *** 0.01 level, ** 0.05 level, * 0.10 level.

Table 4.5a
Probability of Using Parental Care

Variable name	Pre–school-aged children	School-aged children
Family type		
Dual military	0.02	0.03***
Working civilian spouse	0.44**	0.30
Nonworking civilian spouse	0.64***	0.71***
Single military parent^	0.11	0.37
Family Income		
<$25,000	0.11	
<$50,000		0.43**
$25,000 to $49,999	0.28	
$50,000 to $74,999	0.09	0.19
$75,000+^	0.23	0.20
Distance between home and base		
Lives on base^	0.15	0.31
10 miles or less	0.29**	0.37
11–20 miles	0.19	0.27
More than 20 miles	0.16	0.35
Rank		
Officer	0.25 ...	0.27*
Enlisted^	0.18	0.43
Local median income		
25th percentile	0.22	0.26**
75th percentile	0.20	0.35**
Local child-care supply		
25th percentile	0.20**	0.31*
75th percentile	0.11**	0.32*

^ indicates that this is the omitted category in the regression model. For type of child care, DoD CDC is the omitted category for pre–school-aged children only. Formal civilian care is the omitted category for school-aged children. Asterisks reflect that the predicted probability for this category is significantly different from that of the omitted category or that the relationship between the dependent variable and the independent variable is statistically different from zero: *** 0.01 level, ** 0.05 level, * 0.10 level.

coefficient has the opposite interpretation. Because multinomial logistic model coefficients provide little insight regarding the magnitude of the relationships between outcomes and independent variables, in Tables 4.6a and 4.6b we present predicted probabilities for statistically significant variables using these coefficient estimates.

Table 4.6
Child Care Choice for Pre–School- and School-Aged Children

Child-care-choice variable name	Pre–school-aged children		School-aged children	
	Coefficient	Standard error	Coefficient	Standard error
	DoD FCC			
Family has another child aged 13–18 years	−0.2915	1.6906		
Dual military	−0.5113	1.5929		
Working civilian spouse	2.7059	1.7660		
Nonworking civilian spouse	−2.6247**	1.0291		
Work hours vary	−12.1122***	4.3975		
Family income <$25,000	−11.3181***	3.2934		
Family income $25,000 to $49,999				
Family income <$50,000	−11.9235***	3.2349		
Family income $50,000 to $74,999	−2.4581	2.1718		
Lives within 10 miles of base	−3.9350	**1.7902		
Lives 11 to 20 miles from base	−1.6794	1.7391		
Lives >20 miles from base	−9.6802***	3.6544		
Officer	−0.5920	1.1829		
Army	−0.3084	1.2706		
Navy	−44.1423***	5.9953		
Marines				
Navy/Marines	10.3645***	3.7954		
Reserves	0.0149	0.0693		
Median income in local area	−0.5481***	0.1739		
Female unemployment rate	0.0553	0.0369		
Local child-care supply	15.4743***	3.8725		
Constant	−0.2915	1.6906		

Table 4.6
Continued

Child-care-choice variable name	Pre–school-aged children		School-aged children	
	Coefficient	Standard error	Coefficient	Standard error
Formal civilian care				
Family has another child aged 13–18 years			3.6959	3.6523
Dual military	–2.4454*	1.3477	2.4686	2.3031
Working civilian spouse	–2.2699	1.3855	–0.4725	1.5006
Nonworking civilian spouse	–1.9530	1.4813	10.8706***	4.1349
Work hours vary	0.3810	0.8719	–11.7949**	5.3361
Family income <$25,000	–3.7545	2.7488		
Family income $25,000 to $49,999	–3.8617	2.6780		
Family income <$50,000			–9.3324*	4.7988
Family income $50,000 to $74,999	–3.7134	2.5391	–17.6955**	8.3515
Lives within 10 miles of base	2.8967**	1.2502	11.5494**	5.2771
Lives 11 to 20 miles from base	4.2172***	1.6018	12.1264**	5.1806
Lives >20 miles from base	4.8302***	1.5192	19.7617**	9.9599
Officer	–0.0724	2.5614	5.0452	4.4944
Army	0.6332	1.0026	–0.1265	1.2039
Navy	–0.5873	1.1550		
Marines	–45.2791***	8.3972		
Navy/Marines			–0.2892	1.2337
Reserves	4.9034	3.2607	–5.5092**	2.5121
Median income in local area	–0.1685***	0.0762	–0.1041	0.1272
Female unemployment rate	0.0967	0.1210	0.6081	0.4019
Local child-care supply	0.0545	0.0390	–0.0001	0.0218
Constant	5.1342	3.3453	8.0950	6.0770

Table 4.6
Continued

Child-care-choice variable name	Pre–school-aged children		School-aged children	
	Coefficient	Standard error	Coefficient	Standard error
Other care				
Family has another child aged 13–18 years			6.2090*	3.4757
Dual military	–0.9030	1.5145	0.6054	1.8599
Working civilian spouse	–1.0533	1.2547	2.1200	1.4136
Nonworking civilian spouse	0.4960	1.3337	13.3036***	4.0085
Work hours vary	–1.7727*	0.9725	–11.6978***	5.1474
Family income <$25,000	–2.3162	2.9295		
Family income $25,000 to $49,999	–3.5784	2.5473		
Family income <$50,000			–7.4930**	4.8786
Family income $50,000 to $74,999	–3.0629	2.3325	–15.7821**	8.0463
Lives within 10 miles of base	2.4935***	0.8636	11.0908**	4.7101
Lives 11 to 20 miles from base	1.9657	1.2749	13.3349***	4.7201
Lives >20 miles from base	1.9259*	1.0907	20.7033**	9.6421
Officer	–0.2000	2.0464	3.9913	4.2637
Army	1.0560	1.1182	1.6171	1.1001
Navy	0.7498	1.2843		
Marines	–2.1612	1.8617		
Navy/Marines			0.4872	1.3348
Reserves	6.1326**	2.8719	0.2956	1.4043
Median income in local area	–0.1218*	0.0646	–0.1131	0.1385
Female unemployment rate	0.0869	0.1207	0.6577	0.4014
Local child-care supply	0.0424***	0.0136	0.0133	0.0176
Constant	4.1717	3.8784	4.8687	6.3913
$N = 252$	$N = 251$		$N = 194$	
	$F_{(54,431)} = 69.62$		$F_{(34,451)} = 1.81$	
	Prob $> F = 0.0000$		Prob $> F = 0.0041$	

Significance levels: *** 0.01 level, ** 0.05 level, * 0.10 level.

Table 4.6a
Predicted Probability of Using Child Care Options Among Families Using Nonparental Care for Pre–School-Aged Children

Variable name	DoD CDC	DoD FCC	Formal civilian care	Other care
		Family type		
Dual military	0.27	0.19	0.32*	0.22
Working civilian spouse	0.28	0.17	0.35	0.20
Nonworking civilian spouse	0.13	0.38	0.22	0.28
Single military parent^	0.13	0.13	0.58	0.16
		Work hours vary week to week		
Yes	0.28	0.14**	0.43	0.16*
No^	0.15	0.30	0.19	0.36
		Family income		
<$25,000	0.30	0.05***	0.25	0.40
$25,000 to $49,999	0.36	0.09***	0.32	0.23
$50,000 to $74,999	0.34	0.06***	0.31	0.29
$75,000+^	0.02	0.59	0.26	0.13
		Distance between home and base		
Lives on base^	0.33	0.48	0.07	0.18
10 miles or less	0.22	0.17	0.26**	0.34
11–20 miles	0.18	0.09	0.55***	0.18
More than 20 miles	0.13	0.18	0.59***	0.11*
		Rank		
Officer	0.29	0.11***	0.17	0.23
Enlisted^	0.22	0.50	0.36	0.11
		Reservist		
Yes	0.01	0.56***	0.21	0.23**
No^	0.28	0.11	0.41	0.20
		Service		
Air Force^	0.23	0.21	0.37	0.18
Army	0.18	0.13	0.40	0.29
Navy	0.24	0.18	0.25	0.33
Marines	0.64	0.00***	0.00***	0.36

Table 4.6a
Continued

Variable name	DoD CDC	DoD FCC	Formal civilian care	Other care
Local female unemployment rate				
25th percentile	0.21	0.35***	0.28	0.16
75th percentile	0.25	0.11***	0.39	0.26
Local median income				
25th percentile	0.17	0.14	0.44***	0.25*
75th percentile	0.25	0.20	0.33***	0.22*
Local child-care supply				
25th percentile	0.24	0.19	0.35	0.22***
75th percentile	0.22	0.20	0.36	0.23***

^ indicates that this is the omitted category in the regression model. For type of child care, DoD CDC is the omitted category for pre–school-aged children only. Formal civilian care is the omitted category for school-aged children. Asterisks reflect that the predicted probability for this category is significantly different from that of the omitted category or that the relationship between the dependent variable and the independent variable is statistically different from zero: *** 0.01 level, ** 0.05 level, * 0.10 level.

For families with a child aged 0 through 5 years, the first thing we note is that family income plays a significant role in child care choice. Families earning less than $75,000 per year are more than 34 percentage points less likely to use FCC over CDC than are families earning more than $75,000 per year—a finding that accords with our hypothesis that the families who receive larger subsidies (and, hence, pay less) for CDC care are more likely to use that care. We also find that families in which the work hours vary are 14 percentage points less likely to use FCC relative to CDC—surprising, considering that, at least in theory, FCC arrangements are more flexible and may be able to accommodate an unusual work schedule, whereas the CDCs are typically open set hours (e.g., 6 a.m. to 6 p.m.). As our focus groups suggested, it may be that at least some FCC arrangements can be actually less flexible than CDC arrangements. A number of focus group participants indicated that FCC providers are open fewer hours than the CDC.

Proximity to the installation is also an important factor in child care choice. Families living between 11 and 20 miles from the installation are less likely to use FCC than CDC care, compared with families that live on base. Across the board, families living off base are more likely to use formal civilian child-care options over the DoD CDC, and that propensity to use civilian child care increases as the distance from the installation grows. Families who live off base but near to the installation are more likely to use other care options over the CDC. Again, these results are consistent with our hypothesis that proximity to home is an important consideration for families in terms of child care choice, and that families who live off base (and, particularly, those who live far from the installation) are less likely to use DoD-sponsored care options located on base.

Table 4.6b
Predicted Probability of Using Child Care Options Among Families Using Nonparental Care for School-Aged Children

Variable name	All DoD care	Formal civilian care	Other care
Family type			
Dual military	0.23	0.63	0.14
Working civilian spouse	0.24	0.24	0.51
Nonworking civilian spouse	0.04	0.29***	0.67***
Single military parent^	0.29	0.46	0.25
Work hours vary week to week			
Yes	0.36	0.41***	0.23***
No^	0.09	0.54	0.37
Family income			
<$50,000	0.19	0.45*	0.37**
$50,000 to $74,999	0.51	0.27**	0.22**
$75,000+^	0.06	0.65	0.28
Distance between home and base			
Lives on base^	0.52	0.35	0.14
10 miles or less	0.17	0.56**	0.27**
11-20 miles	0.14	0.45**	0.41***
More than 20 miles	0.03	0.53**	0.44**
Reservist			
Yes	0.26	0.13**	0.61**
No^	0.23	0.53	0.24
Family has another child aged 13–18			
Yes	0.12	0.36	0.52*
No^	0.25	0.48	0.27

^ indicates that this is the omitted category in the regression model. For type of child care, DoD CDC is the omitted category for pre–school-aged children only. Formal civilian care is the omitted category for school-aged children.
Asterisks reflect that the predicted probability for this category is significantly different from that of the omitted category: *** 0.01 level, ** 0.05 level, * 0.10 level.

Relative to the Air Force, survey respondents in the Marine Corps were less likely to choose FCC (21 percentage points less likely) or formal civilian-care (37 percentage points less likely) options over CDC care. Reservists were more likely to use FCC and other care options over the CDC. Families living in areas with higher median incomes are less likely to use formal civilian-care options, while families living in areas with a high supply of child care workers are more likely to use formal civilian-care options and other, informal care options as opposed to the CDC. If we assume that the cost of civilian child care is higher in areas in which median incomes are higher, then it appears that military families are willing to use civilian child-care options when those options are available and affordable.

Table 4.6b presents results of the analysis of child care choice for families with school-aged children.

Again, we find a relationship between various family and installation characteristics and child care choice. Families who have another child between the ages of 13 and 18 years are 25 percentage points more likely to use other informal care options relative to those who do not. Most likely, the teenaged children care for the younger children. Families with a civilian spouse who does not work outside the home but who use some form of nonparental care are much less likely to use DoD-run forms of care for their school-aged children than single military parents. Across the board, families living off base are more likely to use formal civilian child-care options and other informal options over the DoD-run child-care options than are families living on base.

CHAPTER FIVE

Conclusions

In this technical report, we have presented the results of our focus groups and survey, and have provided an analysis of the survey results, supplemented by focus group findings. The analysis allowed us to identify factors influencing the use of child care among military families, as well as the installation and family characteristics associated with unmet or poorly met child-care need. A related RAND report (Moini, Zellman, and Gates, 2006) draws on this information to evaluate the DoD's child-care-demand formula.

As suggested in the introduction of this report (Chapter One), DoD is interested in better understanding the demand for child care among military families so that it can more effectively meet the needs of these families. Our analysis provides some conceptual and empirically based insights that should be useful to policymakers.

Child Care Demand Is a Difficult Concept to Analyze in the DoD Context

Although policymakers in DoD and elsewhere often use the term *child care demand,* we have emphasized that the demand for child care is extremely difficult to estimate. Demand for child care cannot be expressed by describing a concrete number of spaces. Rather, it is a relationship between price, features of child care, and the amount of child care that families might wish to consume. In an organization such as the DoD, which subsidizes the cost of care and is involved in the provision of some types of child care, the decisions made by policymakers can be expected to influence how much care parents wish to consume.

In this technical report, we specify four different outcomes that policymakers might be interested in and analyze the factors that are related to those outcomes. The first outcome of interest is *unmet need,* defined as families who report that they would like to use a formal child-care arrangement but are not currently doing so. An analysis of this outcome provides DoD with a measure of how well it is meeting the basic child-care needs of families and which families are better or less well served. A second outcome of interest is *unmet preference,* defined by families who report that the child care option that they are currently using is not their first choice. This may includes families who have unmet need, but also those families whose basic need for child care is being met, just not in the way they might like. The analysis of unmet preference can help DoD understand how child care options could be improved to better meet the needs of military families, and which families appear to be less well served by the current system. A third outcome of interest is whether military families report that they have considered leaving the military due to child care issues. This outcome may be of particular interest to DoD to the extent that it views child care as a means to improve the quality of life of military families and improve retention. Fourth, we consider the child care

51

choices made by military families to understand whether observable characteristics of families and locales are related to the child care choice that families make. This analysis is probably the closest thing to an analysis of child care demand. It can help DoD understand the factors that make families more or less likely to use different types of care and may help DoD better target its child care resources.

We find that there is an important relationship between two of those outcomes: unmet child-care preference and propensity to leave the military. Families that express unmet child-care preference are also more likely to report that child care issues might drive them to leave the military.

Unmet Child-Care Need Is Not Prevalent Among Military Families

Just under 10 percent of military families report unmet child-care need. Although this percentage is low, DoD may be concerned that it is not zero. We found that unmet need is much more prevalent among families with pre–school-aged rather than school-aged children. This finding suggests that while DoD continues to be concerned about providing care for school-aged children, the biggest problem continues to be with caring for pre–school-aged children. Families with a civilian working spouse are more likely to express unmet need, as are families earning less than $50,000 per year. These findings suggest that policies that give dual-military and single parents a preference for DoD-sponsored care may be effective in reducing unmet need among these populations. However, among families with a civilian spouse, low family income may be an outcome of unmet child-care need.

Unmet Preference Is More Common Than Unmet Need

A larger proportion of military families, 22 percent, reported unmet preference for child care. Again, we found a greater prevalence of unmet preference among families with pre–school-aged children. Families have unmet preference for different types of care. Overall, 44 percent of the families who reported unmet preference stated that their preferred form of care is one that is provided by DoD. That means that over half of families expressing unmet preference would like something other than what DoD currently provides. This finding suggests that DoD may need to develop other ways of supporting child care to better meet the child care "demands" of military families.

Child Care Concerns May Influence Retention Decisions

Nearly one-third of survey respondents reported that it is likely or very likely that child care issues would lead them to leave the military. It is important to emphasize that the fact that individuals reported that they are likely to leave the service does not mean that they will act on that sentiment. Further information would be needed to determine whether individuals who express a propensity to leave the service due to child care issues actually do so. Nevertheless, families with pre–school-aged children were much more likely to report a propensity to leave the military than were families with school-aged children.

This difference may be partially due to the fact that the parents of older children tend to be older themselves and to have a longer tenure in and stronger commitment to the military career. Family status appears to have a strong relationship with plans to leave the service. Families with a nonworking civilian spouse are much less likely to express such plans.

Families using CDC care are more likely to express plans to leave the military—a surprising finding in some respects, given that these families receive a large subsidy. In other respects, it is not so surprising. CDC parents often report that they believe CDC care costs too much. Most are unaware of the substantial subsidy they are receiving, and some even believe that the DoD is making a profit from the CDCs.

Dual-Military and Single-Parent Families Experience Challenges

Despite the fact that DoD policy gives special priority to dual-military and single-parent families in terms of accessing DoD-sponsored child-care options, such families are much more likely to report that they plan to leave the military due to child care issues—even though these families are less likely to report unmet need. This may reflect the greater challenges of raising children in the military, either alone or with another military spouse, even when child care is available. It may also reflect the fact that the type of care for which single and dual-military parents receive a preference (CDC care) is the least flexible arrangement and may be least able to accommodate the demands of the military schedule.

Families Living Off Base Are Less Likely to Use DoD-Sponsored Care

The distance between a family's home and the installation is strongly related to the type of child care it uses. Families that live off base are less likely to use DoD-sponsored child-care options, and the propensity to use DoD-sponsored care is lower for families that live farther from base. It appears that many families that live off base do not find DoD-sponsored care, which is typically located on the installation, to be a convenient option. These families do seem to find other options that meet their needs.

It may be that, although DoD-sponsored care is able to meet the needs of many, if not most, families who live on base, those families who live and work on base are less attracted to off-base options if they cannot be accommodated by DoD-sponsored care. This suggests that the housing patterns of military families stationed on a particular installation are an important characteristic for DoD to consider in deciding how to allocate its child care resources.

DoD CDC Users Appear to Have a Weaker Attachment to the Military

The conventional wisdom is that DoD CDC care is the most sought after and convenient type of child care among military families. Certainly, waiting lists are long, and the subsidy provided to families who use this type of care is much larger than the subsidy available for any other type of care. However, our analysis reveals that, controlling for family type, families who use the DoD CDCs are more likely than families who use other care options to report that they are likely to leave the military due to child care issues. Given that the DoD heavily subsidizes care provided in the CDCs, and provides little or no subsidy for other options, DoD may be interested in more fully understanding the attitudes of CDC families.

Local Market Conditions Are Related to the Child Care Choices That DoD Families Make

DoD-sponsored care is an important option for military families; however, it is not the only option. Our analysis reveals that families with pre–school-aged children who live in areas with lower median incomes and families who live in areas with a greater supply of child care workers are more likely to use civilian-sponsored child care than DoD-sponsored care. The relationship between the supply of child care workers and the use of civilian child-care options is obvious.

The relationship between median income and use of civilian-sponsored child care may reflect the implications of differences in cost of living. Since the income of military families does not vary much by locale, military families who live in affluent communities may be less willing or able to pay the market price for civilian child care than military families who live in poorer communities. This finding suggests that characteristics of the local community may be important determinants of the relative need for DoD-sponsored care.

Attention to these issues may help DoD effectively allocate its child care resources.

Results from This Study May Help Inform DoD Policy Decisions Related to Child Care

In a companion report (Moini, Zellman, and Gates, 2006), we apply the results of this study to the question of how DoD characterizes and responds to child care need. That report recommends that DoD consider a broader range of child care outcomes, clearly articulating those that are most important in developing child care policies. We recommend that DoD consider the factors that influence child care outcomes in designing policy responses and suggest that DoD consider providing more options to more fully address need. Such options might include child care vouchers, subsidized spaces in civilian centers, subsidized wraparound[1] care, or support for after-school programs in the community.

DoD recently introduced a new program called "Operation: Military Child Care" that can serve as an example of a type of policy option DoD might want to pursue further. The program seeks to aid active-duty, Reserve, and National Guard families who do not have access to on-base DoD-sponsored care in locating child care and will defray the cost of that care while military members of these families are mobilized or deployed. Clear DoD guidance, combined with a package of policy options that extend beyond creating spaces in DoD-sponsored care, holds promise for better utilizing child care resources to promote DoD goals, increase family choice, and support child well-being.

---

[1] *Wraparound care* is child care that is provided before a CDC or FCC opens and after it closes. CDCs and FCCs typically have standard hours of operation, but military families often have workdays (or have to pull 24-hour shifts) that extend beyond the hours of operation.

Focus Group Summary

This appendix provides a summary of and insights on the need for child care among military families, distilled from recent focus groups. The objective of conducting focus groups with military parents was to learn about the characteristics of child care that parents consider most important, the types and availability of child care on and around installations, and how child care influences career decisions, including the decision to stay in the military. We expected that the results of the focus groups would provide valuable information about child care issues in the military and would inform the design of a survey that would be fielded DoD-wide to gain an in-depth understanding of child care need among DoD families.

Overview of Sites

We conducted 21 focus groups at 8 installations across the country from November 2002 through July 2003. We visited two installations from each service, including Twentynine Palms Marine Corps Base, Camp Pendleton Marine Corps Base, Fort Hood, Fort Meade, Corpus Christi Naval Air Station, Jacksonville Naval Air Station, Mountain Home Air Force Base, and Warner Robins Air Force Base. These bases were selected for focus group sites to provide representation of all the military services and to reflect the variations in socio-economic status of the surrounding community, proximity to urban and rural areas, stringency of state licensing requirements for child care providers, and the ratio of child care centers to state population. These dimensions potentially affect the set of choices parents face when making decisions about child care.

At each site, we contacted the directors of child and youth services for assistance in arranging focus groups with parents who use one or more of four types of care—the child development center (CDC), family child care (FCC), off-base care, or no formal child care. We aimed to have between eight and ten participants in each group, although the actual sizes of the groups varied. We spoke to both mothers and fathers from single-parent and dual-military families, as well as civilians married to military members.

In some cases, parents using different types of care were combined into one focus group to accommodate parents' schedules. Parents using off-base care or no formal child care—a small group—were the most difficult to schedule. And, at a few bases, such parents were unavailable. In general, however, we had good representation of parents using all types of care in each of the services. The focus group interviews followed a structured interview protocol (see Appendix C).

In addition to the focus groups, we conducted interviews with the directors of child and youth services and with the directors of resources and referral and/or family child care at each installation to get an overview of the CDC and FCC availability, impressions of child care need, off-base options for child care, and the programs and policies in place to meet the particular needs of families on the installation.

CDC Parents Appeared to Be Quite Satisfied

Parents who chose to use the CDC instead of other options cited several reasons they felt the DoD CDC on base was the best option for their family, as well as reasons they do not like CDC.

Parents Appreciate the Structure and Security of the CDC

There is a perception that CDCs are cleaner and have more resources than civilian centers or FCCs. Many parents expressed their satisfaction with the CDC facilities and staff, and said they were reassured by the stringent DoD regulations that are often more rigorous than those enforced by the state.

Many parents mentioned the presence of security cameras in the CDC classrooms and the opportunity provided to parents to view their children's activities at any time during the day as a major benefit of CDC care. This monitoring provides parents with a level of comfort about the safety of their children.

Having multiple providers available reassures some parents that if one provider becomes worn out, there are others around to give them a break. One participant said, "There is no telling what family child-care providers who are left alone might do to your child. The CDC lets me go to work and not worry."

Many focus group parents who chose center care viewed it as more reliable than family child care (FCC). If providers at the CDC get sick or must be absent, there are others to fill in, which is not always the case in FCC arrangements.

Many parents like having their child on base near at least one parent. Such proximity allows parents the convenience of being able to easily pick up a child in case of illness or an emergency, as well as the ability to drop in during the workday to check on their child's activities.

CDC Hours of Operation and Curriculum Frustrate Some Parents

Those using the CDC disliked several aspects of care. We should note that the complaints of military parents using CDCs mirror complaints of parents in the civilian sector who use center-based care. Consequently, these complaints should not be viewed as specific to DoD CDCs. Parents complained about hours of operation and the 10-hour-per-day rule, which we discuss in greater detail below.

Parents have mixed feelings about the curriculum at the CDCs. Many would like more-structured teaching because they do not believe the unstructured developmental approach adequately prepares their children for school. Some compared the unstructured approach currently used with the curriculum at civilian centers; one participant said, "The CDC is not pushing her to learn like they did at the civilian center I was at before. For example, there they said, 'This week we are going to learn shapes and you will know this by the end of the week' . . . [at the DoD CDC] they don't test her to see if she got it." The CDC director at one base we visited recognized some parents' dissatisfaction with the CDC approach to learning and was undertaking efforts to educate parents about why the DoD has opted to structure its programs as they do.

Several civilian spouses who participated in the focus groups mentioned the quandary they faced because of the CDC rule that civilian spouses must be working to enroll in the CDC, yet lack of care was what constrained them in searching for work. Some mentioned the challenges they encountered because of this rule when they were forced to quit or were fired from jobs because of schedule constraints imposed when their spouse was deployed (see below for further discussion of spousal employment).

Focus group participants cited the long waiting lists on some bases for certain age groups (particularly infants) as problematic, and several complained about the inconsistent administration of the waiting list. For example, some bases allow children to be put on the list before the family arrives on base, whereas others do not. Also, several participants said that they had to be especially proactive in calling the center each month to check on their waiting-list status or else they might not have gotten in to the CDC. Many people reported that they had to use child care arrangements that they were extremely unhappy with while they were on the waiting list. Other parents were "forced" into other arrangements, such as off-base care or FCC, only to find that they liked them quite well.

Perspectives on FCC Vary Widely

Many focus group participants using FCC homes said they liked the personal attention their children receive from the FCC provider and believe that their children have more interaction with providers and other children in a smaller environment than with center care. They also believe their children are sick less often.

The major problem with FCC homes cited by focus group participants was lack of reliability. When FCC providers or their families get sick, care becomes unavailable and parents must activate backup arrangements that are difficult to use. FCC providers are required to have backup providers who will care for kids in their absence, but these arrangements do not always work in practice. Most often, backup providers are unavailable because their spaces are full. If FCC providers decide to close their doors for any number of reasons, including vacations, spouse deployment, or Permanent Change of Station (PCS), or because they decide to no longer provide care, parents have no recourse and must scramble to find other care arrangements.

Parents Cited Several Reasons for Using Off-Base Care

Parents who were using off-base care reported various reasons for doing so. Overall, these parents were happy with their care arrangement and did not express concerns about quality.

For many, off-base care was a temporary measure to obtain care while the family remained on the waiting list for DoD care. Such parents prefer DoD care for reasons mentioned above.

The other common reason parents use off-base care is because it is less costly, at least in more rural or remote areas. Private providers often allow families to enroll children part-time and to pay only for the number of hours used. Many private providers offer a multichild discount, and they do not require families to pay for child care when the child is on vacation.

Location is also an important consideration for families. For those who live off base, it is often more convenient to use a center off base, close to home—particularly when the family needs a secondary care arrangement (for example, to cover extended hours after the primary arrangement closes). Parents of school-aged children often prefer programs that are close to the child's school. Several parents indicated that the DoD programs will not provide transportation to and from their child's school, which ends up being a substantial barrier to using DoD care.

Some parents sought care in off-base centers because they offered a more academic curriculum and seemed to provide better preparation for school. A few parents with special-needs children said that the DoD centers could not accommodate their child and that they had to seek care off base.

Parental Care Is the Preferred Option for Many Families

We also heard from parents who were not using any formal child care. Many of these parents stated that they felt that it was important to care for their own children at home. In some cases, their adamance extended to a belief in home schooling their children. Parents at Mountain Home AFB said that the public schools in Idaho were terrible; that opinion drove many parents to home school. Several of the children and youth program directors mentioned that they were getting requests for access to the youth center or child care centers for activities for home-schooled children.

Others reported that they were "lucky enough" to have relatives that lived nearby and could provide care. There was an implicit belief, particularly among parents of infants and toddlers, that care by a relative is better than center or family child care. These parents preferred relative care to other types of care.

Some military spouses who were caring for their children reported that they would very much like to work outside the home, but the cost of child care exceeds the amount of money they would earn working. Some of these spouses were frustrated by the lack of good jobs in the local area and/or a lack of affordable child care; others were happy with their decision to take some time off from working outside the home.

Some families manage to care for their children without formal child care, even when both parents work outside the home, by coordinating their work schedules so that one parent is always home.

Focus Group Discussions Highlighted Other Issues and Concerns

Several other issues and concerns about child care emerged across the focus groups. We discuss these issues in the next several subsections.

As Expected, There Were Complaints About the Cost of Child Care

The complaints that military parents expressed about child care are similar to the complaints that working families in the civilian world typically express. The cost of care was an important concern among most focus group participants. Many felt that DoD CDC care was very expensive. Several participants had the impression that the CDCs are making a profit from the child care fees; they seemed to have little knowledge of the amount of DoD subsidy that is provided to run the centers.

Many parents complained about the way the rates are determined, especially the inclusion of Basic Allowance for Housing (BAH) as part of parents' income. Including BAH in the calculation of child care fees made their rates on the sliding-fee scale higher because individuals with children get a larger BAH.

Some participants had the impression that dual-military families pay more for care than do military members with civilian spouses, and felt that it was unfair. There is an impression that individuals with civilian spouses can underreport spousal income.

Family child care is often less expensive, as a percentage of income, for higher-income families than it is for lower-income military members, because providers charge a flat fee rather than use the sliding scale. The flexibility of FCC to accommodate part-time schedules makes it a cheaper alternative for some families that can stagger parents' work schedules. Part-time care is not available in most CDCs. Also, subsidies for infant care in FCCs help offset the cost of the most expensive type of care.

Those with multiple children in the center complain that the rates should be prorated because it gets very expensive for large families. CDC administrators maintain that the cost of providing care is no less for multiple children, so the fees cannot be lowered.

The cost of CDC care influenced some focus group participants to put their children in off-base care or FCC when they would prefer to use the CDC. At other bases, it was exactly the opposite: Some parents preferred an off-base center or FCC providers who could give more-individualized attention, administer medications, etc., but the cost was prohibitive and the CDC became the most feasible option.

Paying to hold a space during deployment and vacation is a burden in the view of many. Some withdraw their children from care in order to avoid paying fees during the time they will be away, if they are reasonably assured that they will be able to get back in.

Lack of Options for Those with Irregular Hours

The most vocal complaints came from parents who worked odd, unusual, or inconsistent work schedules. Most military members are required to work extended hours periodically. Also, there are certain days when the CDC is closed because most of the base is shut down for holidays, but certain military members working in jobs considered "essential" must still report for duty. These families must find alternative forms of care to cover the days that the CDC is not available. One focus group participant at a Marine Corps base we visited said, "A Marine is a Marine 24 hours a day, but the centers are on a 6 a.m.–to–6 p.m. schedule. The FCCs go on leave. What are you supposed to do?"

Parents use various strategies for dealing with this problem. Military members and civilian spouses work with each other, friends, and colleagues to meet the need for care during the hours that care is not available at the CDC. The CDC hours and closures are an especially acute problem for single parents, since they usually lack another adult in the household with whom to share responsibility for the child's care. One participant said, "We do a 'switcheroo' at work with other single parents when they have watch duty. Single parents come together and get to know each other to make the child care arrangements. It is a juggling act." Some families use a combination of family child care and CDC care to cover the amount of care they need, but doing so is costly. Some families use FCC in place of the CDC when they have 24-hour duty, which means they are paying for both CDC care and FCC at the same time.

The most frequently cited benefit of FCC is the flexibility of the hours of operation, including longer hours of daily operation, options for care during extended-duty hours, and part-time-care arrangements, all of which are not possible in the CDC. However, on some bases, FCC was viewed as having less-flexible hours of operation because of unique FCC family situations—for example, one provider's husband wants the FCC kids out of the house before he gets home.

Some bases have extended-duty programs that provide family child care for parents during the hours that the CDC is unavailable. In the Air Force, the Extended Duty Program is funded centrally through the Air Force and provided at no extra cost to families. So far, this program does not seem to be well utilized. Most focus group participants at Air Force bases were not aware of the existence of the program, and those that did know about it were uncomfortable using the care because of the unfamiliarity of those providers.

Another issue about CDC hours that was raised in one of the focus groups was the rule enforced by some CDCs allowing children to be at the center for no more than 10 hours per day. Some focus group participants said that this rule is not flexible enough to meet military schedules, which can be erratic. Instead, it was suggested that a maximum number of hours that children are allowed to be in care should be set by week, because some workdays are much longer than others.

Challenges Facing Families Who Live or Work Far from Base

Some focus group parents reported living a significant distance from the installation, or reported that the civilian spouse was working far from the installation. The most common reason for such a decision was spousal employment opportunities. Second, focus group participants at bases considered remote from urban locations cited the problem of long commutes to areas in which there are better job options for military spouses, especially for educated spouses with professional careers. Such commutes affect child care options and choice, because care arrangements may become untenable when the military spouse deploys or is on a temporary assignment away from home: The location and hours of care might not meet the needs of the spouse commuting several hours per day to a job.

Cost of living was a factor in some locations (e.g., Camp Pendleton, Fort Meade), and issues of public-school quality and neighborhood characteristics came into play. For some of these parents, on-base care was simply not an option, and these parents felt that they were left out of the system.

Other Issues

The overwhelming majority of focus group participants said that child care is a major issue in their decision to stay in the military. Many have considered leaving the service because of child care challenges. Several said that unless child care is taken care of, they cannot concentrate on their jobs. One participant said,

> As a military parent, I feel split right down the middle: half of me is a soldier, and the other half is a mother . . . you can't separate the two. If something is wrong on

one side, it affects the other. Your mind is not on your job if you are worried about the kids.

Because military families move around so much, away from family and social networks, the importance of having good options is vital.

A major challenge that focus group participants named was handling the care of sick children—and dealing with the strict rules governing such care in DoD centers and FCCs. Many parents in the focus groups felt that the rules were excessive and were often enforced without consideration of specific circumstances. An example that several parents cited was when their child was merely teething and had a fever of 99 degrees, and not ill, they were called to pick up the child.

Another rule considered burdensome by some parents is the waiting period of 24 hours that children must be well before returning to the center or FCC. Finally, many parents wish the centers could administer medicines to children. Under the current rules, parents must come in to the center to give medications when needed. This is an enormous inconvenience in some cases. Some would like to see an on-site nurse who would be responsible for the health care of children in the centers.

Many parents are very interested in the idea of creating a mildly ill center, to take care of kids when they are too sick to be with other children but well enough to be away from their parents. Some parents had concerns, however, including the following:

- Bosses would make them use the care, even if they felt they should stay home with the child.
- The child would be exposed to unknown illnesses and might end up sick with something else.
- A child who is sick belongs with Mom or Dad at home, not in a child care center.

Several parents noted that on-base care can cause problems when base access is restricted due to high-terrorist-alert levels. Often, secondary caregivers are not allowed on base during such periods, so they cannot provide the extended care the parent needs after the CDC closes.

Also, parents mentioned a variety of challenges stemming from deployment. For example, the child care arrangement may have worked with the military member's work schedule, but it may not fit well with the schedule of the civilian parent. Hours of operation can become a major concern if the spouse works off base. Single parents reported that they may lose access to care if they have to send their child to live with another relative during a deployment.

Conclusions

Overall, the focus group discussions suggest that both parent satisfaction with and availability of DoD-provided child care vary across installations. While some installations appeared to be meeting the demand for child care during normal working hours, other installations struggle to do so. In particular, the installations that were struggling to provide child care spaces were working very hard to recruit family child-care providers. However, it appeared that the harder an installation was working to recruit family child-care providers, the less satisfied parents were with the FCC provided on base. This difficulty suggests that the supply of FCC providers is not limitless, and additional policies may be needed to expand the provider base.

The focus groups also raise some concerns about whether the structure of DoD child care ignores some important DoD-specific needs by operating and heavily subsidizing a system of child care that provides care primarily during regular-duty hours. However, many military parents, including those who use DoD care, struggle to find care when they have night duty, irregular shifts, weekend exercises, etc. For individuals who have consistently irregular schedules, or rotating shifts, the child care provided by DoD may not be an option at all. In that sense, a failure to provide options that mesh with the military work schedule may be suppressing demand.

Similarly, the nature of services provided limits the usefulness of child care to parents. The unwillingness of CDCs to dispense medications requires parents to take time off work to administer medications. A lack of mildly ill care requires parents to come up with alternative arrangements. Also, the perception that there is a 10-hour-per-day rule may also limit center usefulness.

Despite substantial progress in the military over the past 15 years, parents indicate that it is still challenging to raise children and have a career in the military, particularly for single parents or parents with a spouse who is employed outside the home.

Finally, we found a deep lack of understanding of child care funding issues among military parents. Many parents are suspicious of the child care payment system and believe that DoD is making a profit from child care fees, when, in fact, child care is heavily subsidized. A communication effort could help ameliorate this problem.

Survey Nonresponse Analysis

In this appendix, we present the results of an analysis of survey nonresponse. This analysis uses information we had about sampled individuals to predict the probability that an individual responded to the survey.

The analysis includes the following variables:

Reserve: an indicator variable that takes on a value of 1 if the service member is a member of the Reserves, and 0 otherwise.

Service: A categorical variable indicating an individual's service. Variables included in the model are Army, Navy, and Marines. Air Force is the omitted, or reference, category.

Rank: A categorical variable indicating an individual's rank. We group some ranks due to small sample sizes for any one rank. E-5 is the omitted, or reference, category. The other categories included in the model are E-0–E-3, E-4, E-6, E-7–E-9, O-1–O-2, O-3, O-4, W-1–W-4.

Male: An indicator variable that takes on a value of 1 if the individual is male, 0 if the individual is female.

Race: A categorical variable indicating an individual's race. White is the omitted, or reference, category. Variables included in the model are Black and Other. Other Race includes American Indian, Asian, Native Hawaiian or Pacific Islander, Indian, or Unknown.

Years of service: We included a categorical variable reflecting whether an individual had 0–4, 5–9, or 10 or more years of service. The omitted category is 10 or more years of service.

Education level: We included an indicator variable that takes on a value of 1 if the individual has attained a B.A. degree or higher level of education.

Table B.1 reflects the results of a logit model estimating the probability that an individual responded to the survey as a function of these observable characteristics. Although the explanatory power of the model is not high (Pseudo R-squared of .08), many of the variables are statistically significantly related to response probability. Specifically, women are substantially more likely than men to respond to the survey, as are more highly educated

Table B.1
Survey Nonresponse Analysis

Characteristics of sampled individual	Coefficient
Reserve	−0.228
Army	−0.335***
Navy	−0.092
Marines	−0.271
E-1–E-3	−0.228
E-4	−0.519***
E-6	0.209
E-7+	0.561***
O-1–O-2	0.632**
O-3	0.842***
O-4	0.898***
O-5–O-6	0.987***
W-1–W-4	0.688*
Male	−0.538***
Black	−0.446***
Other Race	−0.122
Years of Service 0–4	−0.187
Years of Service 5–9	−0.181
Bachelor's Degree or Higher Education	0.420***
Constant	−0.412**
	$N = 3,316$
	Pseudo $R^2 = 0.0804$

Significance levels: *** 0.01 level, ** 0.05 level, * 0.10 level.

individuals. Blacks are less likely than Whites to respond. Individuals in the Army are less likely than those in the Air Force to respond. Officers and senior enlisted are more likely to respond to the survey.

We used the results of this analysis to construct nonresponse weights and used weighted data in reporting the results of the survey. However, we are not able to correct for any response bias that may be due to unobservable characteristics (such as deployment status at the time of the survey).

Child-Care Survey Instrument

The authors developed this survey in order to gather information on child care choice, child care use, and family-specific factors that would be expected to influence child care choice and use. The survey instrument was tested at several of the focus group sites and revised on the basis of that feedback.

CARD 01   *5-6/*

RCS-DD-P&R(OT)2168

1-4/   Expiration: 10/31/2006

DATE RCVD: ☐ ☐ ☐ ☐ ☐ ☐   *7-12/*   BATCH ☐ ☐ ☐ ☐   *13-16/*

MILITARY CHILD CARE SURVEY

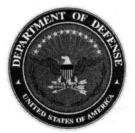

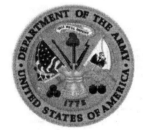

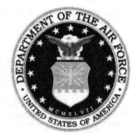

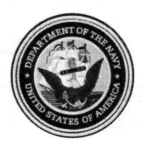

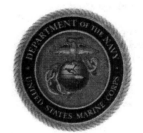

17/

This questionnaire is to be filled out by either or both parents about the child whose name appears on the label.	
If this child does NOT live with you AND you do not participate in any child care decisions, please check here and return this survey in the enclosed self-addressed envelope: [ ]	→ Child's Name Child's Age

RAND Corporation, 1700 Main St., P.O. Box 2138
Santa Monica, CA 90407-2138

Rev 2/19/2004

ABOUT THIS QUESTIONNAIRE

PURPOSE

- The purpose of this survey is to help the Services better understand service members' child care needs, preferences, and problems.

- This survey, being fielded by the RAND Corporation, a nonprofit research institution in Santa Monica, California, and supported by the Office of the Secretary of Defense, is being conducted in coordination with the Army, Air Force, Navy, and Marine Corps and the Defense Manpower Data Center (DMDC) of the Department of Defense.

WHY SHOULD I BOTHER?

- You have been selected at random to represent a larger group of military parents in all four Services. We will combine your responses with the responses of other parents to draw conclusions about the views and experiences of parents overall. We need responses from all types of parents—single parents, dual military parents, as well as military members with civilian spouses.

- While no decisions about you alone will be made based on this survey, survey results will influence policy discussions and may result in changes that affect you as well as other military parents. **If you don't respond, your views and the views of other parents like you will not be considered in military child care policy reviews and changes.**

WILL MY SURVEY RESPONSES BE KEPT PRIVATE?

- YES. **RAND and DMDC will treat your answers as strictly confidential.** Your responses will be combined with information from many other members to report the views and experiences of different types of military parents. Comments may be reported word for word, but never with identifiable information.

- **RAND and DMDC will not release data that could identify you to anyone.** No supervisors or other officials will see your questionnaire, nor will RAND or DMDC release any data that could identify you to anyone in your Service, other Department of Defense agencies, or anyone else, except as required by law.

- We may combine your survey responses with information provided to us by the Department of Defense from your administrative files, such as your military occupational specialty, your duty assignments, your reenlistment status, and so forth. We may also request your participation in a follow-up survey at a future date.

- This study is completely voluntary. There is no penalty if you choose not to respond. However, RAND and the Department of Defense strongly encourage you to participate. If you prefer not to answer a specific questions for any reason, you may just leave it blank.

PRIVACY NOTICE

In accordance with the Privacy Act of 1974 (Public Law 93-579), this notice informs you of the purpose of the survey and how findings will be used. Please read it carefully.

AUTHORITY: 10 United States Code, Sections 136, 1782 and 2358.

PRINCIPAL PURPOSE: Information collected in this survey will be used to assist in formulating policies that affect personnel management, retention, and quality of life for enlisted service members. Reports will be provided to the Secretary of Defense, each Military Service, and the Joint Chiefs of Staff. Results will be used in reports and testimony provided to Congress. Some results may be published by RAND, the Defense Manpower Data Center (DMDC) or professional journals, or reported in manuscripts presented at conferences, symposia, and scientific meetings. In no case will the data be reported or used to identify individual respondents.

DISCLOSURE: Your participation in this survey is voluntary. There is no penalty if you choose not to respond. However, maximum participation is encouraged so that the data will be complete and representative. Your survey instrument will be treated as confidential. Identifying information will be used only by persons engaged in, and for purposes of, the survey research. Only group statistics will be published.

ROUTINE USES: None.

The first group of questions is about the CHILD whose name appears on the survey cover.

- If this child is school-aged and the child's school was in session LAST WEEK, please refer to the child care arrangements you used last week in answering Question 1 about a typical week.

- If this child's school was NOT in session last week, please refer to the LAST WEEK your child's school WAS in session in answering Question 1 about a typical week.

Section 1: Your Child Care Arrangements

1. What child care arrangement do you use the most hours in a typical week during the hours you and/or your spouse are working or attending school? *(If you use more than one source of child care for this child, please check the ONE you use the MOST.)*

   (Check One)   *18-19/*

   DoD Programs:

   ☐1 DoD child development center

   ☐2 DoD home or family child care (FCC)

   ☐3 DoD school age care program

   ☐4 DoD youth center

   ☐5 DoD before or after-school program

   Civilian Programs:

   ☐6 Civilian before or after-school program

   ☐7 Civilian child care center

   ☐8 Civilian family child care

   Parent or Relative Care:

   ☐9 Relative in your home

   ☐10 Relative outside your home

   ☐11 Care provided by mother

   ☐12 Care provided by father

   ☐13 Older sister or brother takes care of child

   ☐14 Child takes care of himself or herself

   Other:

   ☐15 Non-relative in your home

   ☐16 Non-relative outside your home

   ☐17 Other (Specify):

   _____ *20/*

2. How would you rate the quality of care of the child care arrangement you checked in Question 1?

   (Check One)   *21/*

   ☐1 Excellent

   ☐2 Very good

   ☐3 Good

   ☐4 Fair

   ☐5 Poor

3. LAST WEEK, how many hours did you use the child care arrangement you listed in Question 1?

◻◻◻ Number of hours   *22-24/*

4. What was the cost of the child care you listed in Question 1 LAST WEEK or the MOST RECENT WEEK you used it for this child?

$ ◻◻◻ ***(Round to the Nearest Dollar; Enter 0 if you don't pay)***   *25-27/*

5. Using the list below, what were the **FIVE MOST IMPORTANT THINGS** you considered in choosing the child care arrangement you use for the <u>most</u> hours per week? (This is the arrangement you checked in Question 1.)

Logistics:

01. Transportation available
02. Cost
03. Hours of operation
04. Location/convenience
05. Provider could take my child immediately
06. Provider could accommodate all my children
07. Ease of monitoring provider

Nature of Care:

08. Age ranges of other children
09. Available activities
10. Cleanliness
11. Quality of facilities & equipment
12. Academic or school readiness focus
13. Developmental focus

Provider:

14. Child/staff ratio
15. Family environment
16. Religious or cultural environment
17. Familiarity or comfort with provider
18. Provider's philosophy
19. Level of supervision
20. Reliability of care

Other: (Please Specify Below):

21. _____   *28/*

_____

_____

Please enter codes in the boxes below for UP TO FIVE things.

◻◻ 1st Most Important	*29-30/*
◻◻ 2nd Most Important	*31-32/*
◻◻ 3rd Most Important	*33-34/*
◻◻ 4th Most Important	*35-36/*
◻◻ 5th Most Important	*37-38/*

CARD 01   2

6. How satisfied overall are you with the arrangement you checked in Question 1?

   (Check One)   *39/*

   ☐1 Very satisfied

   ☐2 Satisfied

   ☐3 Not completely satisfied

   ☐4 Dissatisfied

   ☐5 Very Dissatisfied

7. If less than very satisfied, what problems do you have with this arrangement? PLEASE PRINT CLEARLY.

   _____ *40/*

   _____

   _____

   _____

8. Thinking about the child care arrangement you checked in Question 1, would you prefer another arrangement?

   (Check One)   *41/*

   ☐1 Yes

   ☐2 No ➔ ***Skip to Question 11, Next Page***

9. If yes, what other child care arrangement would you MOST prefer?

   (Check One)   *42-43/*

   DoD Programs:

   ☐1 DoD child development center

   ☐2 DoD home or family child care (FCC)

   ☐3 DoD school age care program

   ☐4 DoD youth center

   ☐5 DoD before or after-school program

   Civilian Programs:

   ☐6 Civilian before or after-school program

   ☐7 Civilian child care center

   ☐8 Civilian family child care

   Parent or Relative Care:

   ☐9 Relative in your home

   ☐10 Relative outside your home

   ☐11 Care provided by mother

   ☐12 Care provided by father

   ☐13 Older sister or brother takes care of child

   ☐14 Child takes care of himself or herself

   Other:

   ☐15 Non-relative in your home

   ☐16 Non-relative outside your home

   ☐17 Other (Specify):

   _____ *44/*

CARD 01

10. What stops you from using this preferred arrangement for this particular child?

(Check All That Apply)

☐1 Too expensive   *45/*

☐2 Hours not convenient   *46/*

☐3 Location not convenient   *47/*

☐4 Quality not high enough   *48/*

☐5 Lack of availability / No openings right now   *49/*

☐6 Provider can't accommodate my other children   *50/*

☐7 Preferred caretaker (self, relative, sibling) not available to provide care   *51/*

☐8 No reason / No other   *52/*

☐9 Other (Please Specify): _____   *53/*
                                                                                                                54/

11. LAST WEEK, did you use other child care arrangements for this child in addition to the one listed in Question 1? *(Include extra care for weekend work or for 24-hour care, e.g., overnight stays)*

(Check One)   *55/*

☐1 Yes

☐2 No ➔ **Skip to Question 17, Next Page**

12. Please check the **additional** child care arrangements you used for this particular child LAST WEEK.

(Check All That Apply)

DoD Programs:

☐1 DoD child development center   *56/*

☐2 DoD home or family child care (FCC)   *57/*

☐3 DoD school age care program   *-58/*

☐4 DoD youth center   *59/*

☐5 DoD before or after-school program   *60/*

Civilian Programs:

☐6 Civilian before or after-school program *61/*

☐7 Civilian child care center   *62/*

☐8 Civilian family child care   *63/*

Parent or Relative Care:

☐9 Relative in your home   *64/*

☐10 Relative outside your home   *65-66/*

☐11 Care provided by mother   *67-68/*

☐12 Care provided by father   *69-70/*

☐13 Older sister or brother takes care of child *71-72/*

☐14 Child takes care of himself or herself   *73-74/*

Other:

☐15 Non-relative in your home   *75-76/*

☐16 Non-relative outside your home   *77-78/*

☐17 Other (Specify):   *79-80/*

_____

                                                                                     81/

13. How would you rate the average quality of care of the child care arrangements you checked in Question 12?

(Check One)   *7/*

☐₁ Excellent

☐₂ Very good

☐₃ Good

☐₄ Fair

☐₅ Poor

14. Enter the number of hours you used the **additional** child care arrangements you listed in Question 12 LAST WEEK.

☐☐ Number of hours   *8-9/*

15. Enter the cost of the **additional** child care arrangements you listed in Question 12 for this child LAST WEEK.

$ ☐☐☐ *(Round to the nearest dollar; Enter 0 if you don't pay)*   *10-12/*

16. Why did you need more than one child care arrangement for this child LAST WEEK?

(Check All That Apply)

☐₁ My spouse or I worked the night shift   *13/*

☐₂ My spouse or I worked a 24-hour shift   *14/*

☐₃ My spouse or I worked weekends   *15/*

☐₄ My spouse or I worked extended hours   *16/*

☐₅ Unexpected child care need (e.g., child ill, regular care not available, family emergency, school closure)   *17/*

☐₆ My spouse or I attended school   *18/*

☐₇ Other reason (Please Explain): _____   *19/*
20/

17. How long did it take you to find care for the child whose name appears on the survey cover?
(Please answer a and b)

a. After this child was first born (Include search time during pregnancy)		b. When you first moved to this installation	
☐☐ Number of Days, OR	*21-22/*	☐☐ Number of Days, OR	*28-29/*
☐☐ Number of Weeks, OR	*23-24/*	☐☐ Number of Weeks, OR	*30-31/*
☐☐ Number of Months	*25-26/*	☐☐ Number of Months	*32-33/*
☐₁ Not applicable (did not need care after the birth)	*27/*	☐₁ Not applicable (child was born after I arrived at this installation)	*34/*

5

18. Did lack of child care after the birth of your child or when you first moved to this installation keep you or your spouse from:

(Check All That Apply)

☐1 Looking for civilian work   *35/*

☐2 Beginning a civilian job   *36/*

☐3 Reporting for military duty   *37/*

☐4 Attending school   *38/*

☐5 None of the above   *39/*

19. After you found care, did you remain on a waiting list for other preferred child care for this child?

(Check One)   *40/*

☐1 Yes

☐2 No → **Skip to Question 20**

19a.   If yes, how long did it take you to find a child care arrangement that you were comfortable with?

☐☐ # of Days OR	☐☐ # of Weeks OR	☐☐ # of Months
41-42/	*43-44/*	*45-46/*

20. Thinking about the future, how likely is it that child care issues would lead your family to leave the military?

(Check One)   *47/*

☐1 Very likely

☐2 Somewhat likely

☐3 Neither likely or unlikely

☐4 Somewhat unlikely

☐5 Very unlikely

21. To what extent have child care issues had a negative effect on you and your spouse's career advancement and/or affected your choice of assignments?

(Circle one number from 1-6 for each military member and civilian spouse)

	To a Very Great Extent	To a Great Extent	To Some Extent	To a Very Little Extent	Not At All	Not Applicable	
a. Military Member **(FATHER)**:	1	2	3	4	5	6	*48/*
b. Military Member **(MOTHER)**:	1	2	3	4	5	6	*49/*
c. Civilian spouse:	1	2	3	4	5	6	*50/*

Please explain your responses to Questions 20 and 21. PLEASE PRINT CLEARLY.   *51/*

_____
_____
_____
_____
_____

22. Does anyone other than the child's parents or step-parents regularly care for the child?

(Check One)   *52/*

☐₁ Yes ➜ **Skip to Question 25, Next Page**

☐₂ No

23. Why don't you use formal child care arrangements for this child?

_____   *53/*
_____
_____

24. How do you manage without using any type of formal child care for this child?

(Check All That Apply)

☐₁ My spouse or I have flexible work schedules.   *54/*

☐₂ My spouse and I work different shifts.   *55/*

☐₃ One spouse is not working outside the home.   *56/*

☐₄ My child is old enough to take care of himself or herself.   *57/*

☐₅ My child has older brothers or sisters who can take care of him/her.   *58/*

☐₆ One parent is self-employed and works at home.   *59/*

☐₇ Other reason (Please Describe): _____   *60/*
_____   *61/*
_____
_____
_____

Section 2: Most Recent Deployment

25. As a result of the most recent deployment of a military parent for more than 30 days, did your child care arrangement change for the child whose name appears on the survey cover?

    (Check One)   *62/*

    ☐₁ Yes

    ☐₂ No ➜ *Skip to Question 29, Next Page*

    ☐₃ Not applicable / Never deployed ➜ *Skip to Question 29, Next Page*

26. How did your child care arrangement change for this child?

    (Check All That Apply)

    ☐₁ Withdrew from the DoD system   *63/*

    ☐₂ Withdrew from non-DoD care arrangement   *64/*

    ☐₃ Arranged for more care   *65/*

    ☐₄ Civilian spouse left labor force or changed jobs   *66/*

    ☐₅ Child moved elsewhere   *67/*

    ☐₆ Other (Please Specify): _____   *68/*
                                                                                                            69/

27. When the most-recent deployment ended, did you try to return to your pre-deployment child care arrangement?

    (Check One)   *70/*

    ☐₁ Yes

    ☐₂ No

28. When the most-recent deployment ended, how difficult was it to get the child care you needed for the child whose name appears on the survey cover?

    (Check One)   *71/*

    ☐₁ Very difficult

    ☐₂ Difficult

    ☐₃ Somewhat difficult

    ☐₄ A little difficult

    ☐₅ Not at all difficult

Section 3: Your Family Situation

29. What best describes your family situation?

    (Check One)   *72/*

    ☐₁ Single military parent➔ *Skip to Question 37, Page 11*

    ☐₂ Dual military parents ➔ *Skip to Question 37, Page 11*

    ☐₃ Military member, civilian spouse including retired military ➔ *Answer Questions 30-36 below*

30. What is the highest educational attainment of the **civilian spouse**?

    (Check One)   *73/*

    ☐₁ No high school diploma or equivalent

    ☐₂ High school diploma or GED

    ☐₃ Some college

    ☐₄ AA degree

    ☐₅ Bachelor's degree

    ☐₆ More than college degree

31. Which of the following best describes the employment status of the **civilian spouse**?

    (Check All That Apply)

    ☐₁ Full-time employment outside the home   *74/*

    ☐₂ Part-time employment outside the home   *75/*

    ☐₃ Full-time student   *76/*

    ☐₄ Part-time student   *77/*

    ☐₅ Self-employed/working from home   *78/*

    ☐₆ Family or home child care provider   *79/*

    ☐₇ Looking for work   *80/*

    ☐₈ Not employed outside the home   *81/*

    ☐₉ Retired   *82/*

32. How many hours per week does the **civilian spouse** work or attend classes?

    ☐☐☐   Number of hours   **(Enter 0 if neither working nor attending school)**   *83-85/*

> **THESE QUESTIONS SHOULD BE ANSWERED IF THE FAMILY INCLUDES A CIVILIAN SPOUSE.**
> **OTHERS SKIP TO QUESTION 37, PAGE 11**

33. Does the **civilian spouse** usually work or attend classes the same or fixed hours every week, or does his/her hours vary from week to week, such as rotating from days to evenings or nights? *(If the civilian spouse has more than one job, please answer for the job where he/she works the __most__ hours.)*

    (Check One) *7/*

    ☐1 Fixed/same hours

    ☐2 Hours vary from week to week

    ☐3 Don't know ☐4 Not applicable (not working)

34. Where does the **civilian spouse** work for the most hours per week?

    (Check One) *8/*

    ☐1 At the child development center on base

    ☐2 Other job on base

    ☐3 Off base

    ☐4 At home as a family or home child care provider

    ☐5 Self-employed in another business

    ☐6 Other (Please Specify): _____ *9/*

    ☐7 Not applicable (attending school or not working)

35. If the **civilian spouse** is not employed outside the home or attending school full-time, is it due to lack of child care options? *10/*

    ☐1 Yes

    ☐2 No

    ☐3 Not applicable, civilian spouse is employed or in school full-time

36. Please tell us if you agree or disagree with the following statements about **civilian spouse** employment.

    (Circle one number from 1-5 for each statement)

	Strongly Agree	Agree	Neither Agree or Disagree	Disagree	Strongly Disagree	
a. Job opportunities in the local area are limited.	1	2	3	4	5	*11/*
b. Better paying jobs require a long commute.	1	2	3	4	5	*12/*
c. Job opportunities in the local area do not make use of the skills of the civilian spouse.	1	2	3	4	5	*13/*

Section 4: For All Families

37. Do(es) the military parent(s) have a **civilian** job in addition to the military job? *(If dual military parents, record answer for both the father <u>and</u> the mother.)*

   a. Military Member **(FATHER):** ☐₁ Yes ☐₂ No ☐₃ Not Applicable / Father not in the military *14/*

   b. Military Member **(MOTHER):** ☐₁ Yes ☐₂ No ☐₃ Not Applicable / Mother not in the military *15/*

38. In total, **including both military and any paid civilian work**, how many hours do(es) the military parent(s) work during a normal WEEK? If none, enter "0" in the boxes for that parent.

   a. Military Member **(FATHER):** [|] Number of hours <u>per week</u> on military & civilian jobs *16-18/*

                                      ☐₁ Not Applicable / Father not in military   *19/*

   b. Military Member **(MOTHER):** [|] Number of hours <u>per week</u> on military & civilian jobs *20-22/*

                                        ☐₁ Not Applicable / Mother not in military   *23/*

39. Are these hours worked the same every week or do they vary from week to week?

   a. Military Member **(FATHER):**   ☐₁ Hours the same every week   *24/*

                                           ☐₂ Hours vary from week to week

                                           ☐₃ Not Applicable / Father not in military

   b. Military Member **(MOTHER):**   ☐₁ Hours the same every week   *25/*

                                           ☐₂ Hours vary from week to week

                                           ☐₃ Not Applicable / Mother not in military

40. In the LAST FOUR WEEKS, how many times did a parent **arrive late for work or leave early** because of a problem with your child care arrangement (e.g., a sick child or an unscheduled school closure) for the child whose name appears on the survey cover? *(Answer separately for each military member and civilian spouse.)*

   a. Military Member **(FATHER)** was late for work or left early due to child care problems:

     [|] # times in past 4 weeks *26-27/* OR ☐₁ Not Applicable / Father not in the military   *28/*

   b. Military Member **(MOTHER)** was late for work or left early due to child care problems:

     [|] # times in past 4 weeks *29-30/* OR ☐₁ Not Applicable / Mother not in the military   *31/*

   c. **Civilian Spouse** was late for work or left early due to child care problems:

     [|] # times in past 4 weeks *32-33/* OR ☐₁ Not Applicable / Don't have a civilian spouse *34/*
                                                                or spouse does not work

41. In the LAST FOUR WEEKS, did any family member miss at least a day of work or school because of a problem with your child care arrangement (<u>including</u> unscheduled school closure) for the child whose name appears on the survey cover? *(Answer separately for each military member and civilian spouse.)*

    a. Military Member **(FATHER):** ☐₁ Yes ☐₂ No ☐₃ Not Applicable / father not in military   *35/*

    b. Military Member **(MOTHER):** ☐₁ Yes ☐₂ No ☐₃ Not Applicable / mother not in military *36/*

    c. Civilian Spouse: ☐₁ Yes ☐₂ No ☐₃ Not Applicable / no civilian spouse   *37/*

42. Who cared for the child whose name appears on the survey cover the last time your regular child care was not available?

(Check All That Apply)

☐₁ Does not apply; never happened   *38/*

☐₂ Military member stayed or went home   *39/*

☐₃ Civilian spouse stayed or went home   *40/*

☐₄ Military member (mother or father) took child to work   *41/*

☐₅ Civilian spouse took child to work   *42/*

☐₆ Relative watched child   *43/*

☐₇ Neighbor or friend watched child   *44/*

☐₈ Child watched self   *45/*

☐₉ Hired sitter   *46/*

☐₁₀ Older child stayed home   *47-48/*

☐₁₁ Regular provider arranged for substitute care   *49-50/*

☐₁₂ Other (Please Specify): _____   *51-52/*
  53/

☐₁₃ Don't know   *54-55/*

43. In the last four weeks, was the child whose name appears on the survey cover ever sick on a work day?

☐₁ Yes   *56/*

☐₂ No

44. What did you do the last time this child was sick on a work or school day?

(Check All That Apply)

☐1 Took child to regular arrangement   *57/*

☐2 Took child to provider who accepts sick children   *58/*

☐3 Military member stayed or went home   *59/*

☐4 Civilian spouse stayed or went home   *60/*

☐5 Military member took child to work   *61/*

☐6 Civilian spouse took child to work   *62/*

☐7 Relative watched child   *63/*

☐8 Neighbor/friend watched child   *64/*

☐9 Child watched self   *65/*

☐10 Hired sitter   *66-67/*

☐11 Older child stayed home   *68-69/*

☐12 Other (Please Specify): _____   *70-71/*
                                                                          72/

☐13 Don't know   *73-74/*

45. Do you live on a military installation?

(Check One)   *75/*

☐1 Yes → *Skip to Question 48, Next Page*

☐2 No

46. If no, approximately how far away from the installation do you live?

☐☐☐ Miles   *76-78/*

47. Why do you live off of the military installation?

(Check All That Apply)

☐1 No on-base family housing available   *79/*

☐2 Spousal employment   *80/*

☐3 Housing is cheaper   *81/*

☐4 Housing is better quality   *82/*

☐5 Wanted to purchase a home   *83/*

☐6 Community characteristics (e.g., better schools)   *84/*

☐7 Other (Please Specify): _____   *85/*
                                                                          86/

CARD 04   5-6/
1-4/

48. How many children are living with you now?

(**Please answer for the most recent or current accompanied tour.**)

☐☐ Number of children   *7-8/*

49. Please list the first name (or initials) AND date of birth of each of your dependents age 18 and under and indicate whether this child lives with you. Start with the child who is listed on the cover of this questionnaire.

First name or initials	Lives with you		Date of Birth (MM/DD/YYYY)
	YES	**NO**	
a. _____	☐1	☐2 *9/*	☐☐/☐☐/☐☐☐☐ *10-17/*
b. _____	☐1	☐2 *18/*	☐☐/☐☐/☐☐☐☐ *19-26/*
c. _____	☐1	☐2 *27/*	☐☐/☐☐/☐☐☐☐ *28-35/*
d. _____	☐1	☐2 *36/*	☐☐/☐☐/☐☐☐☐ *37-44/*
e. _____	☐1	☐2 *45/*	☐☐/☐☐/☐☐☐☐ *46-53/*
f. _____	☐1	☐2 *54/*	☐☐/☐☐/☐☐☐☐ *55-62/*
g. _____	☐1	☐2 *63/*	☐☐/☐☐/☐☐☐☐ *64-71/*
h. _____	☐1	☐2 *72/*	☐☐/☐☐/☐☐☐☐ *73-80/*

50. What is the rank of the highest-ranking military member in this family?

(**Check One Category Box**)

Enlisted Grades:

☐E-1   ☐E-2   ☐E-3   ☐E-4   ☐E-5   ☐E-6   ☐E-7   ☐E-8   ☐E-9   *81-82/*

Officer Grades:

☐O-1   ☐O-2   ☐O-3   ☐O-4   ☐O-5   ☐O-6 and above

Warrant Officer Grades:

☐W-1   ☐W-2   ☐W-3   ☐W-4

51. What was your <u>total</u> family income **IN 2003** BEFORE TAXES?

INCLUDE:

- All earned income (BEFORE TAXES) including wages, salaries, tips, long-term disability benefits, combat pay and voluntary salary deferrals, retirement or other pension income before deductions for taxes or social security.

- Quarters subsistence and other allowances appropriate for the rank and status of military or civilian personnel whether received in cash or in kind. For dual military members include the BAH II of the senior member only. Include anything else of value, even if not taxable, that was received for providing services.

DO NOT INCLUDE:

- Cost of living allowance (COLA) received in high cost areas, alimony and child support, temporary duty allowances or reimbursements for educational expenses.

(Check One)

☐₁ Less than $ 25,000   *83/*

☐₂ $ 25,000 – $ 49,999

☐₃ $ 50,000 – $ 74,999

☐₄ $ 75,000 – $ 99,999

☐₅ $ 100,000 or more

52. What are the total annual earnings of the **civilian spouse** (if applicable) in 2003 BEFORE TAXES?

(Check One)

☐₁ Less than $ 12,500   *84/*

☐₂ $ 12,500 – $ 24,999

☐₃ $ 25,000 – $ 36,999

☐₄ $ 37,000 – $ 49,999

☐₅ $ 50,000 or more

☐₆ Not applicable. I don't have a civilian spouse.

☐₇ Civilian spouse did not work outside the home.

53. What are your total current child care expenditures for the child whose name appears on the survey cover?

$ ☐ , ☐☐☐ *(Round to the nearest dollar)*   *85-88/*

Per: *(Check One)*

☐₁ Week

☐₂ Month   *89/*

54. What are your total current expenditures for child care for <u>all</u> dependent children living with you including the child whose name appears on the survey cover? *(Do not include private school tuition for school age children, but do include the cost of before- and after-school care.)*

$ ☐ , ☐☐☐ *(Round to the nearest dollar)*   *7-10/*

Per: *(Check One)*

☐1 Week

☐2 Month   *11/*

55. For a child the age of the child whose name appears on the survey cover, how does the cost of off-base center care compare with DoD center care in the area in which you are now living?

(Check One)   *12/*

☐1 More expensive than DoD center care

☐2 The same as DoD center care

☐3 Less expensive than DoD center care

☐4 Don't know

56. For a child the age of the child whose name appears on the survey cover, how does the cost of off-base family child care compare with DoD home or family child care here?

(Check One)   *13/*

☐1 More expensive than DoD family child care

☐2 The same as DoD family child care

☐3 Less expensive than DoD family child care

☐4 Don't know

57. How do the costs of DoD home or family child care compare with DoD center care?

(Check One)   *14/*

☐1 DoD family child care is more expensive than DoD center care

☐2 DoD family child care is the same as DoD center care

☐3 DoD family child care is less expensive than DoD center care

☐4 Don't know

58. Will your provider care for the child whose name appears on the survey cover when he/she is sick?

(Check One)   *15/*

☐1 Yes → *Skip to Question 59*

☐2 No

58a.   If no, if your child was sick, would you be willing to pay an extra amount for care when the regular provider wouldn't accept the child (equivalent to the same amount you currently pay daily)?

(Check One)   *16/*

☐1 Yes

☐2 No

59. Who completed this questionnaire?

(Check One)   *17/*

☐1 Active duty military member (father)

☐2 Active duty military member (mother)

☐3 Civilian Spouse of active duty military member

☐4 Both parents

☐5 Someone else

Who? _____   *18/*

Continue on Next Page

Section 5: Questions about Children Aged 6-12

60. Is the child whose name appears on the survey cover currently attending school in grades 1-8?

(Check One) *19/*

☐₁ No, child is too young. ***You are finished!***

☐₂ No, child is being homeschooled. ➔ ***Please answer Questions 61 - 72***

☐₃ Yes, child is enrolled in grades 1-8. ➔ ***Please answer Questions 61 - 72***

Summer Care for Children Aged 6-12

61. Please check all child care arrangements you used <u>last summer</u> for the child whose name appears on the survey cover.

(Check All That Apply)

☐₁ DoD Summer camp program *20/*

☐₂ Civilian summer camp program *21/*

☐₃ Community recreation program, swimming pool, or supervised playground *22/*

☐₄ School activities program *23/*

☐₅ Civilian day care center *24/*

☐₆ DoD home or family child care (FCC) *25/*

☐₇ Civilian family child care *26/*

☐₈ Cared for by an older brother or sister *27/*

☐₉ Stayed with another relative (other than a brother or sister, e.g., grandparent) *28/*

☐₁₀ Stayed with a neighbor or a friend *29-30/*

☐₁₁ Parental care *31-32/*

☐₁₂ Took care of him / herself *33-34/*

☐₁₃ Other (Please Specify): _____ *35-36/*
37/

62. How satisfied are you with the arrangement you used <u>last summer</u> for the most hours per week for the child whose name appears on the survey cover?

(Check One) *38/*

☐₁ Very satisfied

☐₂ Satisfied

☐₃ Not completely satisfied

☐₄ Dissatisfied

☐₅ Very Dissatisfied

63. If less than very satisfied, what problems do you have with this arrangement? PLEASE PRINT CLEARLY.

39/

_____

_____

64. Thinking about the arrangement you used <u>last summer</u> for the most hours weekly for the child whose name appears on the survey cover, would you have preferred another arrangement?

☐1 Yes   *40/*

☐2 No → **Skip to Question 67, Next Page**

65. If yes, what other arrangement would you have preferred?

(Check One)   *41-42/*

☐1 DoD vacation camp program

☐2 Civilian vacation camp program

☐3 Community recreation program, swimming pool or supervised playground

☐4 School activities program

☐5 Civilian day care center

☐6 DoD home or family child care (FCC)

☐7 Civilian family child care

☐8 Cared for by an older brother or sister

☐9 Stayed with another relative (other than a brother or sister, e.g., grandparent)

☐10 Stayed with a neighbor or a friend

☐11 Parental care / took time off

☐12 Took care of him / herself

☐13 Other (Please Specify):

43/

_____

_____

66. What stopped you from using this preferred arrangement?

(Check All That Apply)

☐1 Too expensive   *44/*

☐2 Hours not convenient   *45/*

☐3 Location not convenient   *46/*

☐4 Quality not high enough   *47/*

☐5 Lack of availability: no openings   *48/*

☐6 Provider couldn't accommodate my other children   *49/*

☐7 Preferred caretaker (self, relative, sibling) not available to provide care *50/*

☐8 Other (Please Specify): _____   *51/*
                                                                               52/
☐9 No reason   *53/*

Care during School Breaks and Holidays (During the School Year)

67. Please check all arrangements you used to care for the child whose name appears on the survey cover during the most recent school break or holiday (<u>other than summer</u>).

    (Check All That Apply)

    ☐₁ DoD vacation camp program   *54/*

    ☐₂ Civilian vacation camp program   *55/*

    ☐₃ Community recreation program or
       supervised playground   *56/*

    ☐₄ School activities program   *57/*

    ☐₅ Civilian day care center   *58/*

    ☐₆ DoD home or family child care (FCC) *59/*

    ☐₇ Civilian family child care   *60/*

    ☐₈ Cared for by an older brother or sister   *61/*

    ☐₉ Stayed with another relative (other than a
       brother or sister, e.g., grandparent)   *62/*

    ☐₁₀ Stayed with a neighbor or a friend   *63-64/*

    ☐₁₁ Parental care / took time off   *65-66/*

    ☐₁₂ Took care of him / herself   *67-68/*

    ☐₁₃ Other (Please Specify):   *69-70/*
                                                 71/
    _____

68. How satisfied were you with the child care arrangement you used during the most recent school break or holiday (<u>other than summer</u>) for the most hours per week for the child whose name appears on the survey cover?

    (Check One)   *72/*

    ☐₁ Very satisfied

    ☐₂ Satisfied

    ☐₃ Not completely satisfied

    ☐₄ Dissatisfied

    ☐₅ Very Dissatisfied

69. If less than very satisfied, what problems do you have with this arrangement? PLEASE PRINT CLEARLY.

    _____ *73/*

    _____

    _____

    _____

70. Thinking about the child care arrangement you used during the most recent school break or holiday (<u>other than summer</u>) for the most hours weekly for the child whose name appears on the survey cover, would you have preferred another arrangement?

    (Check One)   *74/*

    ☐₁ Yes

    ☐₂ No ➔ ***You are finished!***

CARD 05   20

71. If yes, what other child care arrangement would you have preferred?

(Check One)   *75-76/*

☐₁ DoD vacation camp program   ☐₈ Cared for by an older brother or sister

☐₂ Civilian vacation camp program   ☐₉ Stayed with another relative (other than a
                                                         brother or sister, e.g., grandparent)
☐₃ Community recreation program, swimming
     pool, or supervised playground   ☐₁₀ Stayed with a neighbor or a friend

☐₄ School activities program   ☐₁₁ Parental care / took time off

☐₅ Civilian day care center   ☐₁₂ Took care of him / herself

☐₆ DoD home or family child care (FCC)   ☐₁₃ Other (Please Specify):

☐₇ Civilian family child care   _____ *77/*

72. What stopped you from using this preferred arrangement?

(Check All That Apply)

☐₁ Too expensive   *78/*

☐₂ Hours not convenient   *79/*

☐₃ Location not convenient   *80/*

☐₄ Quality not high enough   *81/*

☐₅ Lack of availability: no openings   *82/*

☐₆ Provider couldn't accommodate my other children   *83/*

☐₇ Preferred caretaker (self, relative, sibling) not available to provide care   *84/*

☐₈ Other (Please Specify): _____   *85/*
                                                                          86/
☐₉ No reason   *87/*

THANK YOU FOR COMPLETING THIS SURVEY!!

Please place your completed survey in the envelope provided and mail it to the RAND Corporation.

No Postage Needed!

88-89/

90/

References

Allison, P., "Discrete-Time Methods for the Analysis of Event Histories," *Sociological Methodology,* Vol. 13, 1982, pp. 61–98.

———, *Event History Analysis: Regression for Longitudinal Event Data,* Thousand Oaks, Calif.: Sage Publications, 1984.

Anderson, P., and P. Levine, "Child Care and Mothers' Employment Decisions," in D. Card and R. Blank, eds., *Finding Jobs: Work and Welfare Reform,* New York: Russell Sage Foundation, 2000, pp. 420–462.

Blau, D. M., *The Child Care Problem: An Economic Analysis,* New York: The Russell Sage Foundation, 2001.

Blau, D. M., ed., *The Economics of Child Care,* New York: Russell Sage Foundation, 1991.

Blau, D. M., and A. P. Hagy, "The Demand for Quality in Child Care," *Journal of Political Economy,* Vol. 106, No. 1, 1998, pp. 104–147.

Buddin, R., Carole R. Gresenz, Susan D. Hosek, Marc N. Elliott, and Jennifer Hawes-Dawson, *Evaluation of Housing Options for Military Families,* Santa Monica, Calif.: RAND Corporation, MR-1020-OSD, 1999.

Campbell, N. D., J. Appelbaum, K. Martinson, and E. Martin, *Be All That We Can Be: Lessons from the Military for Improving Our Nation's Child Care System,* Washington, D.C.: National Women's Law Center, 2000.

Chipty, T., "Economic Effects of Quality Regulations in the Day-Care Industry," *AEA Papers and Proceedings,* Vol. 85, No. 2, 1995. pp. 419–424.

Chiuri, M. C., "Quality and Demand of Child Care and Female Labour Supply in Italy," *Labour,* Vol. 14, No. 1, 2000, pp. 97–118.

Connelly, R., D. Degraff, et al., "If You Build It, They Will Come: Parental Use of On-Site Child Care Centers," *Population Research and Policy Review,* Vol. 21, 2002, pp. 241–273.

Gates, Susan M., Cassandra Guarino, Lucrecia Santibañez, and Bonnie Ghosh-Dastidar, with Abigail Brown and Catherine Chung, *Career Paths of School Administrators in North Carolina: Insights from an Analysis of State Data,* Santa Monica, Calif.: RAND Corporation, TR-129-EDU, 2004.

Gordon, R., and L. Chase-Lansdale, "Availability of Child Care in the United States: A Description and Analysis of Data Sources," *Demography,* Vol. 38, No. 2, 2001, pp. 299-316.

Hausman, Jerry, and D. McFadden, "Specification Tests for the Multinomial Logit Model," *Econometrica,* Vol. 52, 1984.

Hofferth, S. L., D. D. Chaplin, et al., "Choice Characteristics and Parents' Child-Care Decisions," *Rationality and Society,* Vol. 8, No. 4, 1996. pp. 453–495.

Hofferth, S. L., and D. A. Wissoker, "Price, Quality, and Income in Child Care Choice," *The Journal of Human Resources,* Vol. XXVII, No. 1, 1991, pp. 70-111.

Hosek, James R., Beth J. Asch, C. Christine Fair, Craig W. Martin, and Michael G. Mattock, *Married to the Military: The Employment and Earnings of Military Wives Compared with Those of Civilian Wives,* Santa Monica, Calif.: RAND Corporation, MR-1565-OSD, 2002.

Johansen, Anne S., Arleen A. Leibowitz, and Linda J. Waite, *The Importance of Child-Care Characteristics to Choice of Care,* Santa Monica, Calif.: RAND Corporation, RP-582, 1997.

Kisker, Ellen, and Rebecca Maynard, "Quality, Cost, and Parental Choice of Child Care," in D. Blau, ed., *The Economics of Child Care,* New York: Russell Sage Foundation, 1991.

Kozaryn, L., "DoD, Services Work to Expand Child Care," American Forces Information Service, 2000. Available online at http://www.dod.gov/news/Aug2000/n08312000_20008312.html.

Lakhani, H., and E. Hoover, "Child Care Use, Earnings, and Retention Desires of Wives of Employees—U.S. Army Officers' Study," *Journal of Economic Psychology,* Vol. 18, 1997, pp. 87–110.

Macro International, Inc. *1999 Family Child Care Research Project Report and Recommendations,* Calverton, Md., 1999.

Michalopoulos, C., P. K. Robins, et al., *A Structural Model of Labor Supply and Child Care Demand,* Madison, Wisc.: University of Wisconsin–Madison Institute for Research on Poverty, 1991.

Moini, J., G. L. Zellman, and S. M. Gates, *Providing Child Care to Military Families: The Role of the Demand Formula in Defining Need and Informing Policy,* Santa Monica, Calif.: RAND Corporation, MG-387-OSD, 2006.

National Academy of Public Administration, *Accessibility and Affordability: A Study of Federal Child Care,* Washington, D.C.: Center for Human Resources Management, 1997.

National Association for the Education of Young Children, *Accreditation Criteria and Procedures of the National Academy of Early Childhood Programs,* Washington, D.C., 1991.

Newell, C. E., P. Rosenfeld, R. N. Harris, and R. L. Hindelang, "Reasons for Nonresponse on U.S. Navy Surveys: A Closer Look," *Military Psychology,* Vol. 16, No. 4, 2004, pp. 265–276.

Powell, L., "Joint Labor Supply and Childcare Choice Decisions of Married Mothers," *The Journal of Human Resources,* Vol. XXXVII, No. 1, 2002, pp. 106–128.

Queralt, M., and A. D. Witte "Estimating the Unmet Need for Services: A Middling Approach," *Social Services Review,* December 1999, pp. 524-559.

———,"Influences on Neighborhood Supply of Child Care in Massachusetts," *Social Services Review,* March 1998, pp. 17–46.

U.S. Department of Defense, *The Potential Demand for Child Care Within the Department of Defense and a Plan to Expand Availability,* A Report to Congress, Washington, D.C.: Office of the Secretary of Defense, Force Management and Personnel, July 1992.

———, "Child Development Programs," memorandum, Washington, D.C., January 19, 1993.

———, Office of Family Policy, "Need for Child Care Spaces by Service," memorandum, Washington, D.C., March 2000.

U.S. Government Accountability Office, *Military Child Care: Extensive, Diverse, and Growing,* Washington, D.C.: GAO-HRD-89-3, 1989.

U.S. Inspector General, U.S. Department of Defense, *Report of Inspection on Military Service Child Care Programs,* Washington, D.C., September 1990.

Van Horn, M. L., S. Ramey, et al. "Reasons for Child Care Choice and Appraisal Among Low-Income Mothers," *Child & Youth Care Forum,* Vol. 30, No. 4, 2001, pp. 231–249.

Zellman, G. L., and Susan M. Gates, *Examining the Cost of Military Child Care,* Santa Monica, Calif.: RAND Corporation, MR-1415-OSD, 2002.

Zellman, G. L., and A. S. Johansen, *Examining the Implementation and Outcomes of the Military Child Care Act of 1989,* Santa Monica, Calif.: RAND Corporation, MR-665-OSD, 1998.

Zellman, G. L., A. S. Johansen, L. Meredith, and M. Selvin, *Improving the Delivery of Military Child Care: An Analysis of Current Operations and New Approaches,* Santa Monica, Calif.: RAND Corporation, R-4145-FMP, 1992.

Zellman, G. L., A. S. Johansen, and J. Van Winkle, *Examining the Effects of Accreditation on Military Child Development Center Operations and Outcomes,* Santa Monica, Calif.: RAND Corporation, MR-524-OSD, 1994.